ATLAS OF THE CELLULAR STRUCTURE OF THE HUMAN NERVOUS SYSTEM

Strange, is it not? that of the myriads who
Before us pass'd the door of Darkness through
Not one returns to tell us of the Road,
Which to discover we must travel too.

Omar Khayyam (11th century)

The contemplation of things as they are,
without error or confusion, without
substitution or imposture, is in itself a
nobler thing than a whole harvest of
invention.

Francis Bacon (1605)

ATLAS OF THE CELLULAR STRUCTURE OF THE HUMAN NERVOUS SYSTEM

Harold Hillman
David Jarman

Unity Laboratory of Applied Neurobiology,
University of Surrey, Guildford, Surrey, England

ACADEMIC PRESS

Harcourt Brace Jovanovich, Publishers
London   San Diego   New York
Boston   Sydney   Tokyo   Toronto

ACADEMIC PRESS LTD.
24/28 Oval Road,
London NW1 7DX

United States Edition published by
ACADEMIC PRESS INC.
San Diego, California 92101-4311

British Library Cataloguing in Publication Data
Hillman, H. (Harold) 1930-
    Atlas of cellular structure of the human nervous system.
    1. Man. Nervous system. Anatomy
    I. Title   II. Jarman, D.
    611.8

ISBN 0-12-348770-6

Filmset by Oxprint Ltd , Oxford
Printed in Hong Kong

CONTENTS

This book is dedicated to our wives,
Elizabeth and Jean.

PREFACE

The great microscopist and cytologist, J. R. Baker, wrote: 'Every cytological investigation should start, if possible, with the study of the living cell' (Baker, 1958). With pleasing exceptions, such as blood vessels in the web of toes, peripheral nerves *in situ* and sympathetic ganglia, this is rarely possible in the living animal, because the optical conditions for light microscopy are not optimal. Observations on tissue culture would be attractive, but, unfortunately, cells change in culture and their appearances are highly sensitive to the conditions of incubation. Therefore, the nearest one can approach the appearance of living cells is to dissect them out using minimal unnatural reagents, and try to observe them before their structure changes, or they become infected.

Study of unfixed human nervous tissue requires access to material from biopsy or from post mortems. Material from the former sources is hard to obtain, and samples from most parts of the central nervous system are not available. Therefore, in this atlas, most of the material is post mortem from human beings. Of course, some of the patients had been dead for 1–3 days before the post mortems, and undoubtedly autolysis will have occurred during this time. However, it is worth noting that: (i) this is a drawback of any human neuropathological study; (ii) as far as we are aware, no one has shown that morphological changes do occur shortly after death in the elements of the central nervous system; (iii) our practice was to discard tissues in which bacteria or fungi could be seen; (iv) we always compared the appearances of the human post-mortem specimens with those of the same structures from freshly killed rabbits, rats, guinea-pigs, lambs and mice. There were no differences between the same structures in the human brains and those in these mammals, except that we did not see lipofuscin in the central nervous systems of animals. Sometimes, when tissues such as retinas or median nerves were not obtainable from human beings, only animal tissues could be used; (v) most of our samples were from middle aged or old human beings, because children and young adults rarely came to post mortem.

In this atlas, we have attempted to make accurate observations on the building materials of the nervous system, rather than on its connections or physiology. Our philosophy has been that the structures speak for themselves, so that our comments are confined to drawing readers' attention to particular structural features and their incidence.

The early pioneers of microscopy, such as van Leeuwenhoek, Fontana, Swammerdam, Malpighi, Purkinje, Remak, Ehrenberg, and Valentin, examined tissues without the addition of fixatives. Fixatives had been used earlier to stop post-mortem changes, but were not widely employed until histological techniques were developed in the second half of the 19th century. The kinds of observations in the earlier literature on unstained cells of the central nervous system were no longer reported after the introduction of histological procedures, and are now rare in modern publications.

Tellyesniczky in 1898 made the first systematic investigations on the effects of staining procedures on the appearances and dimensions of tissue by light microscopy. He was followed by Ross, Baker, Frontera, Gersh, Kushida, Lodin, Cammermeyer and many others. They found that during staining procedures, whether or not they included freezing, the whole tissue shrank, each organelle not necessarily shrinking equally. Shrinkage occurred mainly during fixation, dehydration, and between dehydration and embedding or mounting. The apparent spaces seen around stained neurons were a graphic example of this phenomenon. The widely held belief that the embedding or mounting media reinflated the tissue components to their previous volumes turned out not to be the case (see Appendix, p. 205).

The following chemical effects could also change the appearance of the tissue: (i) precipitates can be formed in the extracellular fluid, the cytoplasm and the axoplasm, firstly, as a consequence of fixation, secondly, from the dehydration of tissues previously containing 60–80 per cent water, and thirdly, when salts of heavy metals, such as silver, osmium, tungsten, lead, etc., react with the proteins and lipids of the tissue; (ii) the large volume of the reagents compared with that of the tissues results in extraction of water and solvent-soluble components, some of them structural. For example, fixatives extract proteins; ethanol and acetone extract lipids.

Since Stilling and Wallach in 1842 introduced serial sections, it has been appreciated that the size, shape or presence of any cell or organelle cannot be assessed from a single section.

The techniques of teasing and microdissection go back to van Leeuwenhoek in the 17th century and were used in this century by Gray, Heilbrunn, the Chambers (father and son) and Hyden. Further, the observation of the fine structure of unfixed cells, previously pursued by bright field, dark ground and polarizing microscopy, was much enhanced by the invention of phase contrast microscopy by Zernike in 1934.

Hyden in Sweden in the 1960s studied the neurons of the Deiters' nucleus of rabbit using this approach, but — as far as we can find — no attempts have been made before to examine all main elements in the mammalian (including human) nervous system, under these conditions. We would be pleased to enter into discussion or correspondence with anyone who has made similar observations.

Many of the historical references are taken from Clarke and O'Malley (1968).

ACKNOWLEDGEMENTS

We are most grateful to the Handicapped Children's Aid Committee of London and to Dr D. Horrobin of Scotia Pharmaceuticals for supporting this work. Mr K. Shaughnessy and Mr J. Darbey of the Audio Visual Aids Unit of the University of Surrey took the colour macrographs. Dr R. Ainsworth and Mr R. Smythe kindly obtained the tissue for us. Mr E. Rosen, FRCS, from Manchester was good enough to supply us with the micrographs of the fundus. Mr A. V. Dodge, former President of the Quekett Microscopical Club, helped us much with the photography and the microscopy.

Miss P. Gunter, of Zeiss Oberkochen Ltd. at Welwyn Garden City, permitted us to use the laser scanning microscope. Mr M. J. Walker, of Stafford, took some flash photographs of our neurons, and Mr L. V. Martin, OBE, former President of the Quekett Microscopical Club, used his Hoffman modulation contrast to look at the structure of the nucleolus. Dr Susan Hall, of the Department of Anatomy, Guy's Hospital, London, and Cambridge University Press gave us permission to reproduce the micrograph of the mouse sciatic nerve. We extend our thanks to all these individuals.

LIST OF FIGURES

Section 3 Cerebral cortex

Section 7 Cranial nerves and retina

Section 8 Peripheral nerves

Section 9 Pituitary, pineal and adrenal glands

METHODS
USED

Most of the observations were made on human brains obtained at post mortem. The patients had been dead for 1–3 days, and had died from non-neurological causes. Their ages ranged from 46 to 95 years. The specimens were not fixed. They were put into plastic bags and taken to the Unity Laboratory of Applied Neurobiology of the University of Surrey within 20 minutes of their excision.

The human brains were initially cut into coronal sections and kept unfixed at 4°C. The slabs were photographed as soon as possible in natural colour.

When human tissues were not available, nervous tissue was taken from lambs which had died during birth and from adult rabbits, rats, guinea-pigs and mice killed by exposure to an overdose of ether. The brains, spinal cords, retinas, cranial nerves, ganglia and peripheral nerves were excised, and the specimens were teased and photographed, usually on the same day but sometimes up to 3 days later. In the latter cases they were placed in specimen bottles in an atmosphere saturated with water vapour, and stored in the refrigerator at 4°C.

Pieces of brain or spinal cord were cut into transverse sections and placed on the stage of a Zeiss zoom dissecting microscope, with magnification from 20 to 200 times. They were bathed in 150 mm NaCl solution (saline) to which about 1 mg methylene blue per 50 ml saline was added to show up the neuron somas and the general topography of the tissue. After this had been established, a small piece about 2 mm, by 2 mm, by 0.05–0.1 mm thick was cut with iris scissors, a scalpel blade, or a fine syringe needle. It was placed in saline in a parallel-walled chamber (Sartory *et al.*, 1971). This was made by cutting a circular hole in double-sided non-water-soluble tape, about 2 cm by 2 cm square, which was stuck on to a microscope slide. The masking tape was left on the upper surface, and a drop of saline was placed in the circle to receive the tissue. The masking tape was removed, and a standard cover slip 0.17 mm thick was placed over the specimen with minimum pressure (Hillman, 1986a).

The small unteased pieces of tissue were observed with minimal teasing under less than optimal conditions to establish the appearances of the cells and nerve fibres *in situ* and to find out whether any appearances in the subsequently teased or microdissected tissues were artefacts produced by the teasing or microdissection itself. This became crucial, for example, when viewing varicosities on fibres and droplets in white matter, which other authors have thought to have resulted from manipulations.

Individual neurons and pieces of neuroglia were isolated by hand by the technique originally described by Hyden (1959), and detailed more recently (Hillman, 1986a). Neuron somas were dissected out by hand, using mounted stainless steel wires 30 μm or 70 μm in diameter, or tungsten wires 150 μm in diameter, brought to a point by the method of Dossel (1966). The somas were transferred on the wire to a drop of saline solution containing no methylene blue, in a parallel-walled chamber. Using the dissecting microscope, a small group of somas, clumps of neuroglia, myelinated fibres, or droplet or varicose fibres, could be placed under direct vision on any part of the slide. They were so isolated that they could be viewed optimally and photographed by phase contrast microscopy.

The specimens were then examined using a Zeiss research microscope and Neofluar objectives, with 6.3, 16, 40, 63 or 100 times magnification and numerical apertures of 0.20, 0.40 and 0.75, 0.9 and 1.3, respectively. Sometimes, two polars were used, when the objects observed were thought to be birefringent. A Zeiss Ikon Icarex 35 camera and Kodak Technical Pan Film 2415 were used, and calibration was performed using a stage micrometer, with 10 μm divisions. All photographs were printed on Ilford Multigrade III paper. Ektachrome 160 was used for colour.

In all cases, the appearances of all elements seen in the human specimens were the same, although often larger than those in the animal specimens studied, except that lipofuscin granules were seen in human but not in animal brains. However, it must be said that most tissues originated from mature human beings and young adult animals. All the appearances of the neurons, neuroglial fibres, granules and droplets observed are reported.

Nearly all tissues were examined fresh by phase contrast microscopy but, nowadays, neurons and glial cells are often identified by their fluorescence on addition of monoclonal antibodies to neurofilament polypeptide or to glial fibrillary acidic protein (GFAP), respectively. Therefore, these antibodies have been used on some identified cells by the method of Debus *et al.* (1983).

Briefly the tissues were fixed in acetone, 5 per cent acetic acid in ethanol, or in buffered paraformaldehyde for 5 minutes at room temperature. They were washed three times with phosphate buffered saline (PBS), the surplus PBS was drawn off, and 50 μl fetal calf serum was left on the cells for 20 minutes. The excess fetal calf serum was removed at room temperature, and 50 μl of the monoclonal antibody, anti-GFAP or anti-neurofilament 200 kD protein, was pipetted on to the preparation; it was left in a moist atmosphere for 12 hours at 4°C. It was washed three times with PBS at room temperature, the surplus PBS was removed, and 50 μl anti-mouse-IgG-FITC (fluorescein isothiocyanate) antibody was pipetted on to it, and left for 1 hour at room temperature, in a moist atmosphere in the dark. The antibodies were supplied by Boehringer Mannheim. The preparation was then washed three times with PBS, and mounted in a PBS/glycerol mixture (Citifluor AF1). The slides were sealed with nail varnish. At no time were the tissues allowed to dry out.

The slides were viewed with a Leitz Dialux 20 fluorescent microscope, using the epifluorescent mode and phase contrast objectives, with 16 or 40 times magnification and numerical apertures of 0.45 and 0.7, respectively. The photographs were taken with an Olympus OM2N camera and Ecktachrome 400 colour film.

SECTION
1

COLOUR MACROGRAPHS
OF THE BRAIN

Views of the intact brain
Sections of the cerebrum and the cerebellum

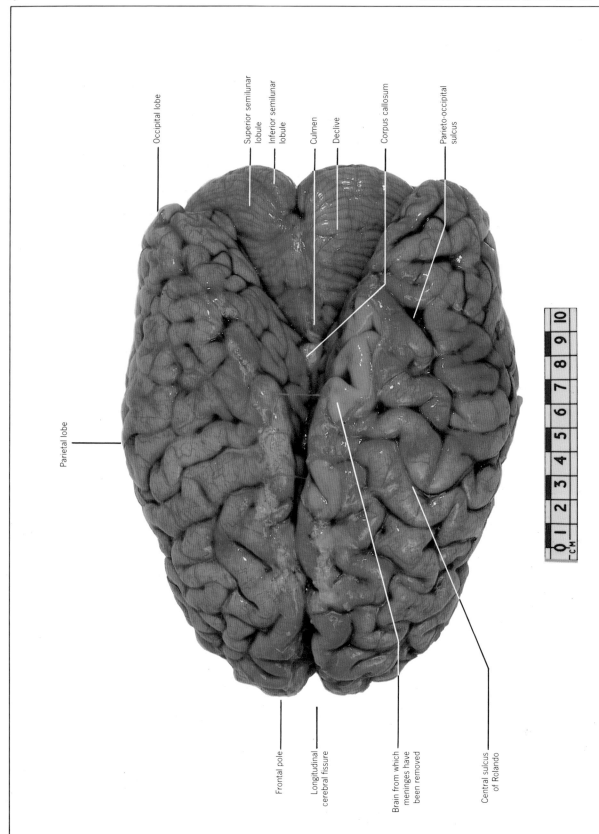

Occipital lobe

Superior semilunar lobule

Inferior semilunar lobule

Culmen

Declive

Corpus callosum

Parieto-occipital sulcus

Parietal lobe

Frontal pole

Longitudinal cerebral fissure

Brain from which meninges have been removed

Central sulcus of Rolando

Figure 1 Superior view of the brain of a 74-year-old man (× 0·67).

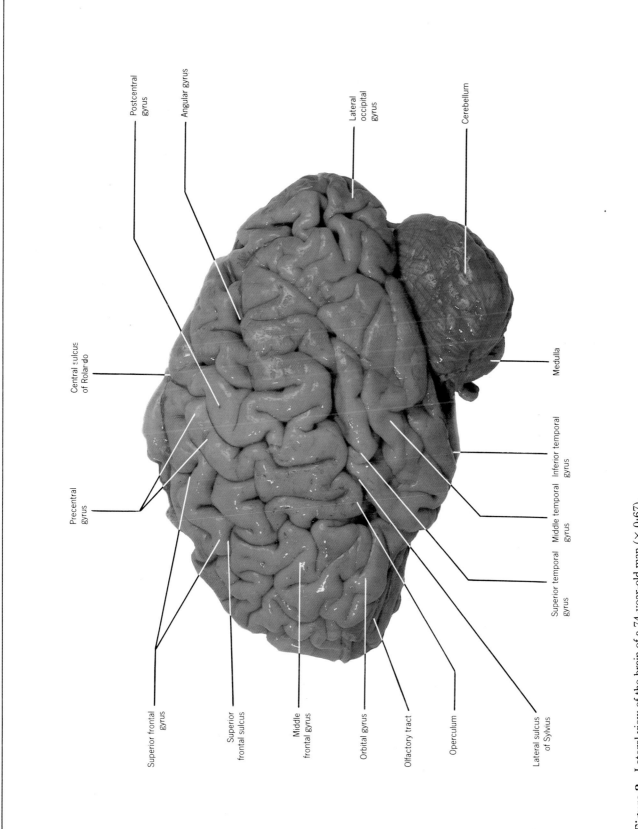

Figure 2 Lateral view of the brain of a 74-year-old man ($\times$ 0·67).

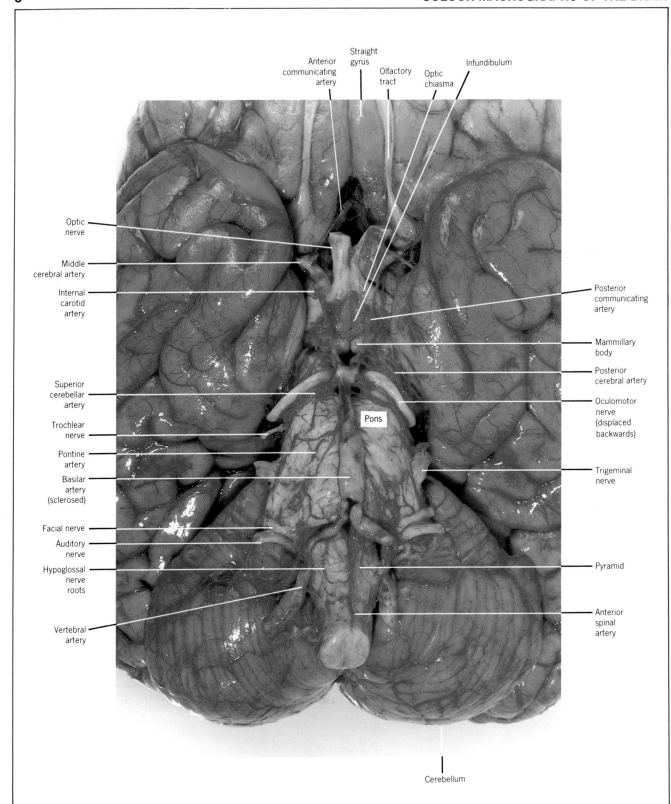

Figure 3 Inferior view of the brain of a 74-year-old man to show some of the cranial nerves. The oculomotor nerve should be pointing forwards (× 1).

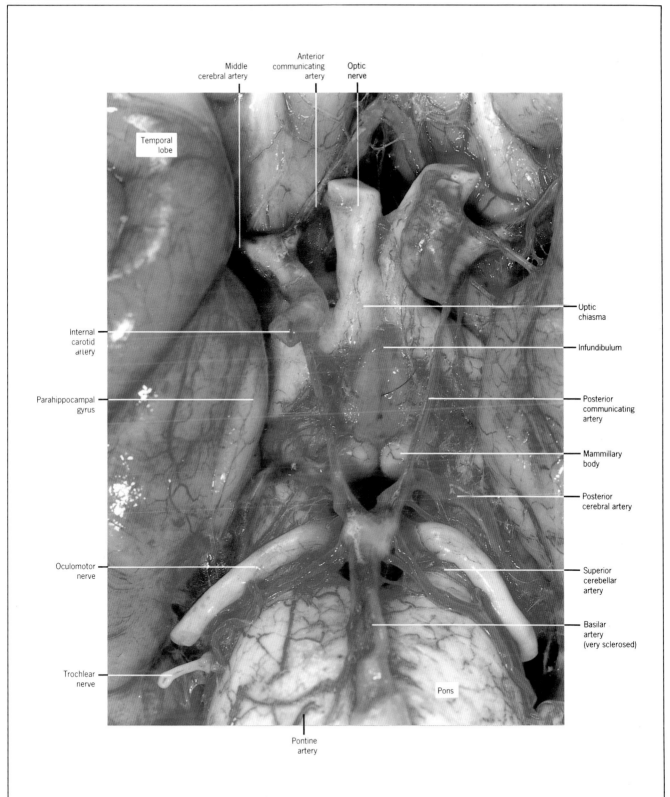

Figure 4 Inferior view of the brain of a 74-year-old man to show the circle of Willis. The sclerosis of the basilar artery is pathological (× 2·5).

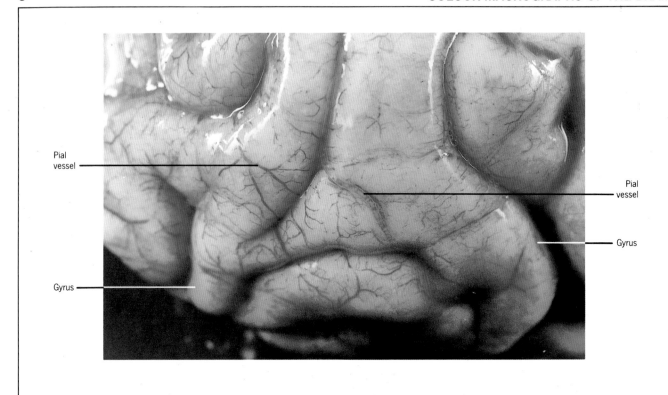

Pial vessel

Pial vessel

Gyrus

Gyrus

Figure 5 Pial vessels on the surface of the cortex (× 3·5).

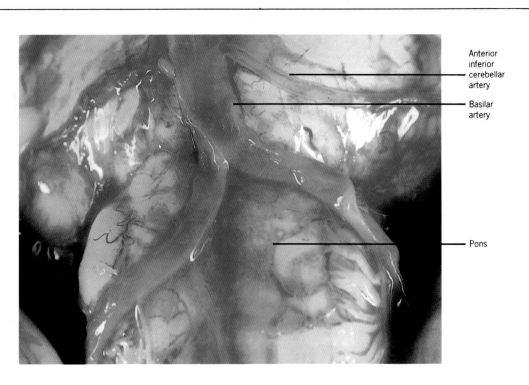

Anterior inferior cerebellar artery

Basilar artery

Pons

Figure 6 Ventral view of the pons, showing two vertebral arteries joining to become the basilar artery, which leads to the circle of Willis (× 3·5).

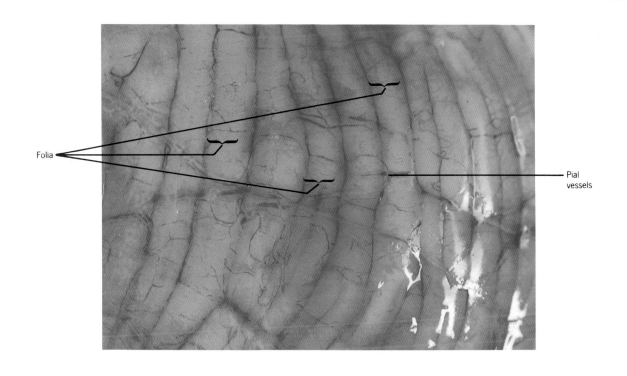

Figure 7 The cerebellum to show the folia and the pial blood vessels (× 3·5).

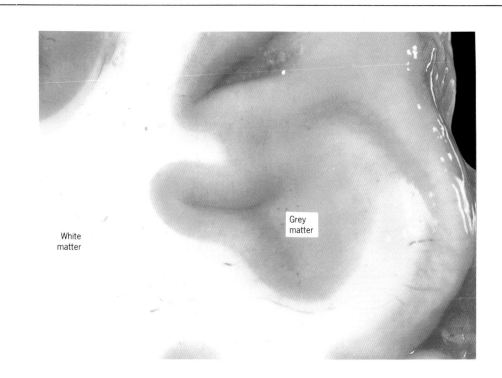

Figure 8 The frontal lobe, showing the white and grey matter, whose colour is light brown in the unfixed state (× 3·5).

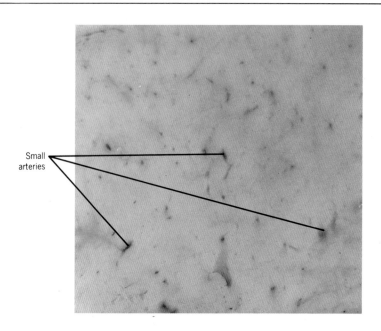

Figure 9   The white matter of the insula to show the distribution of small arteries (× 3·5).

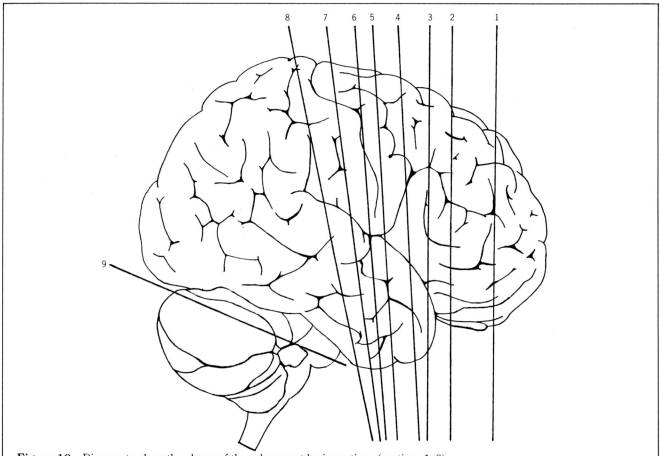

Figure 10   Diagram to show the planes of the subsequent brain sections (sections 1–9).

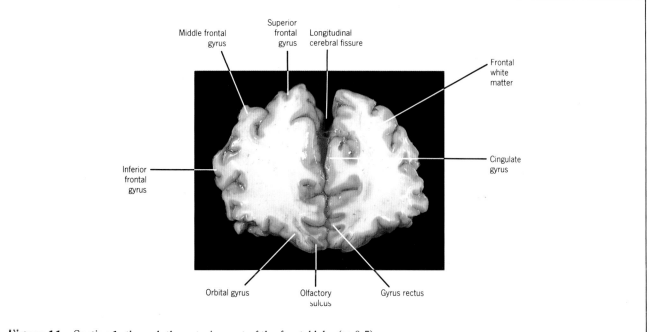

Figure 11 Section 1, through the anterior part of the frontal lobe (× 0·5).

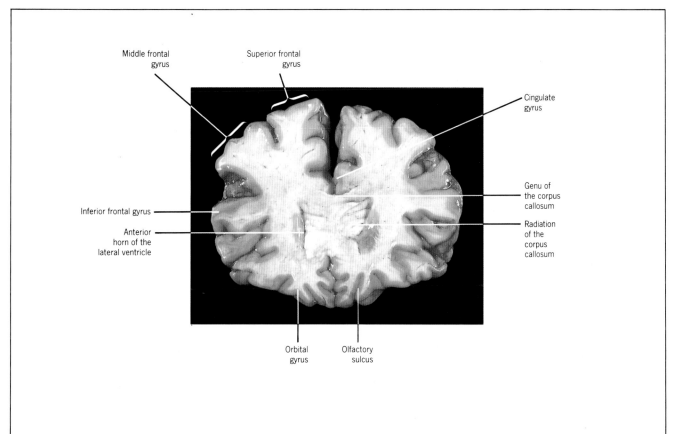

Figure 12 Section 2, through the frontal lobe to show the genu of the corpus callosum and the anterior horns of the lateral ventricle (× 0·5).

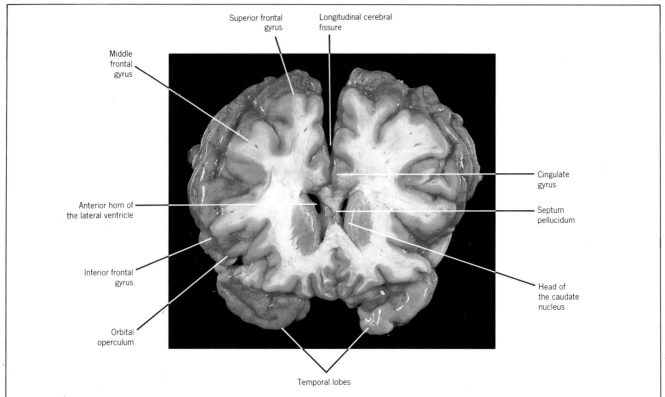

Figure 13   Section 3, through the frontal lobe and the head of the caudate nucleus. The temporal lobes can be seen below (× 0·5).

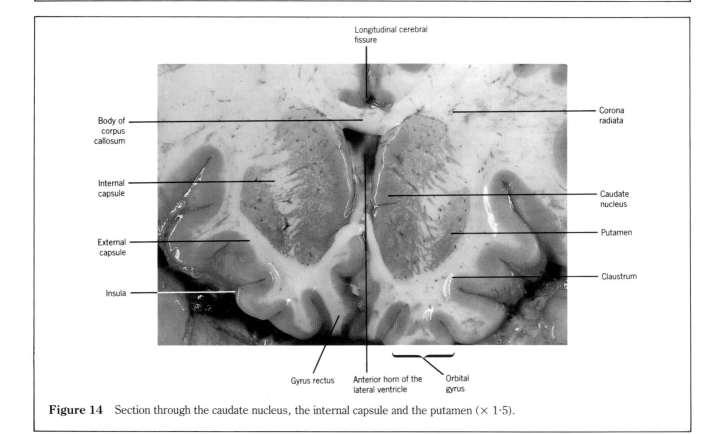

Figure 14   Section through the caudate nucleus, the internal capsule and the putamen (× 1·5).

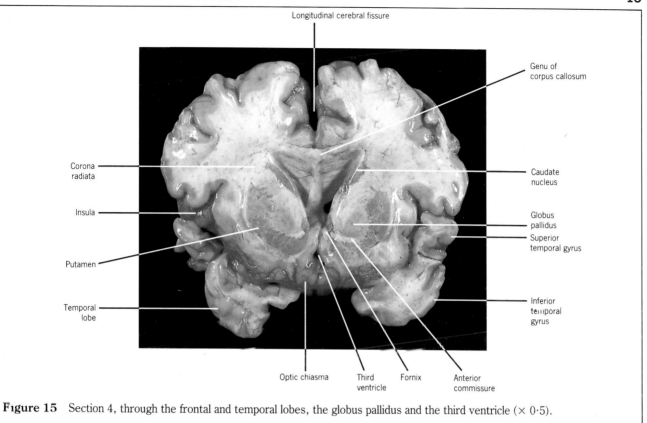

Longitudinal cerebral fissure

Genu of corpus callosum

Corona radiata

Caudate nucleus

Insula

Globus pallidus

Superior temporal gyrus

Putamen

Temporal lobe

Inferior temporal gyrus

Optic chiasma

Third ventricle

Fornix

Anterior commissure

Figure 15   Section 4, through the frontal and temporal lobes, the globus pallidus and the third ventricle (× 0·5).

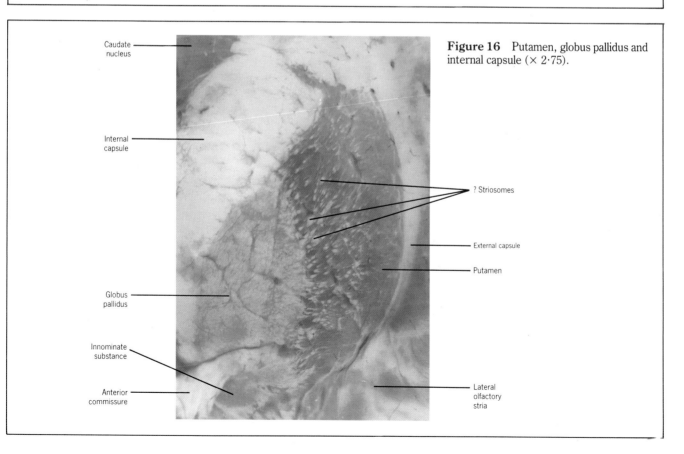

Caudate nucleus

Figure 16   Putamen, globus pallidus and internal capsule (× 2·75).

Internal capsule

? Striosomes

External capsule

Putamen

Globus pallidus

Innominate substance

Anterior commissure

Lateral olfactory stria

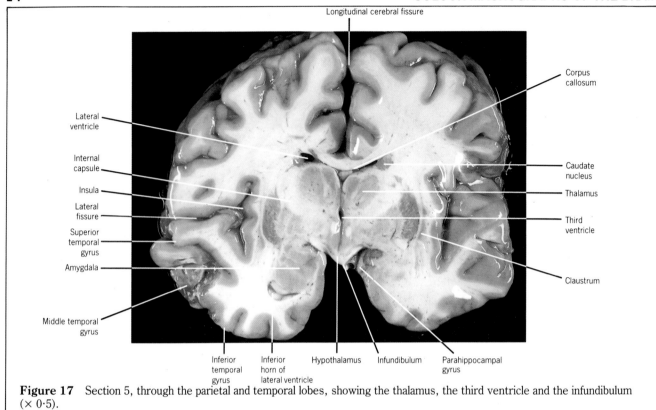

Figure 17 Section 5, through the parietal and temporal lobes, showing the thalamus, the third ventricle and the infundibulum (× 0·5).

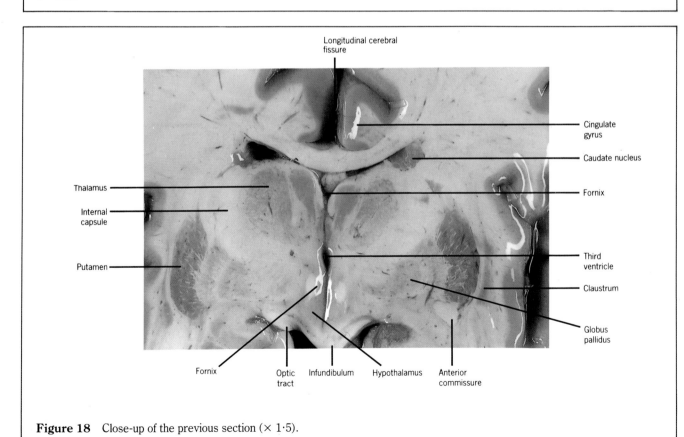

Figure 18 Close-up of the previous section (× 1·5).

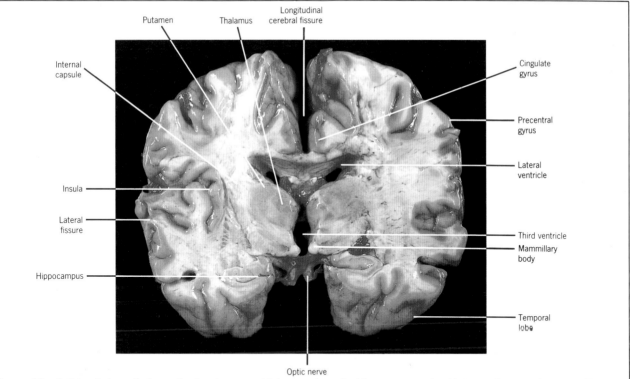

Figure 19 Section 6 through the parietal and temporal lobes to show the hippocampus, the third ventricle and the mammillary bodies (× 0·5).

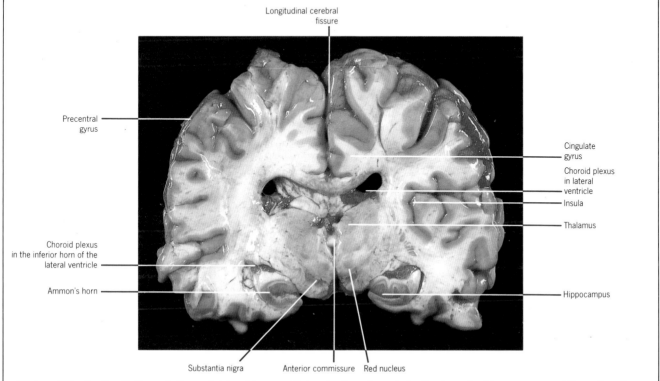

Figure 20 Section 7, through the parietal and temporal lobes to show the substantia nigra, the hippocampus and the red nucleus (× 0·5).

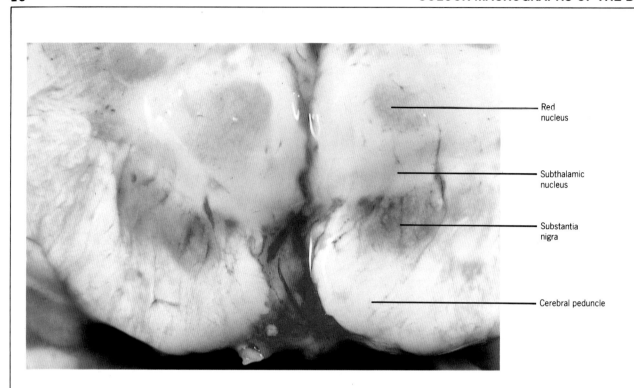

Red
nucleus

Subthalamic
nucleus

Substantia
nigra

Cerebral peduncle

Figure 21   Close-up of the previous figure (× 3·5).

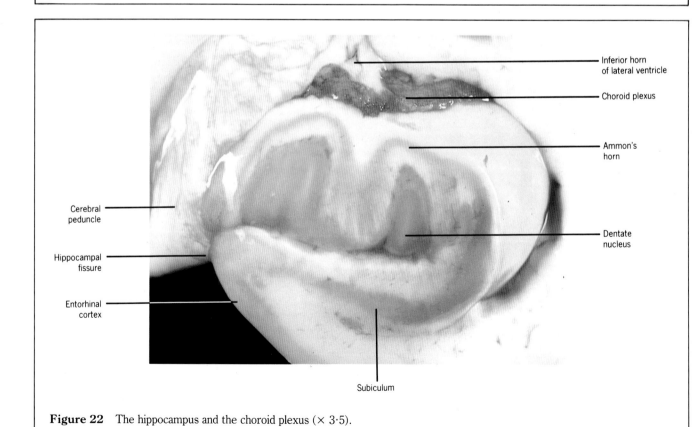

Inferior horn
of lateral ventricle

Choroid plexus

Ammon's
horn

Cerebral
peduncle

Dentate
nucleus

Hippocampal
fissure

Entorhinal
cortex

Subiculum

Figure 22   The hippocampus and the choroid plexus (× 3·5).

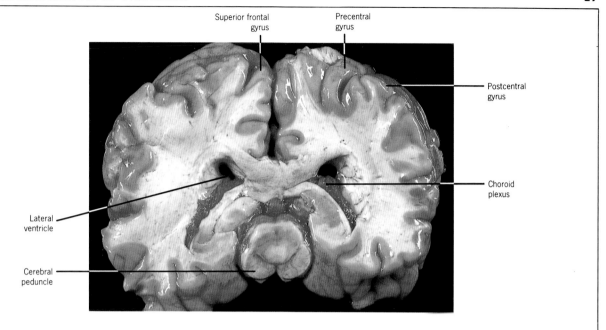

Superior frontal gyrus

Precentral gyrus

Postcentral gyrus

Choroid plexus

Lateral ventricle

Cerebral peduncle

Figure 23 Section 8, through the parietal and temporal lobes, to show the pineal gland, the midbrain and the pons (× 0·5).

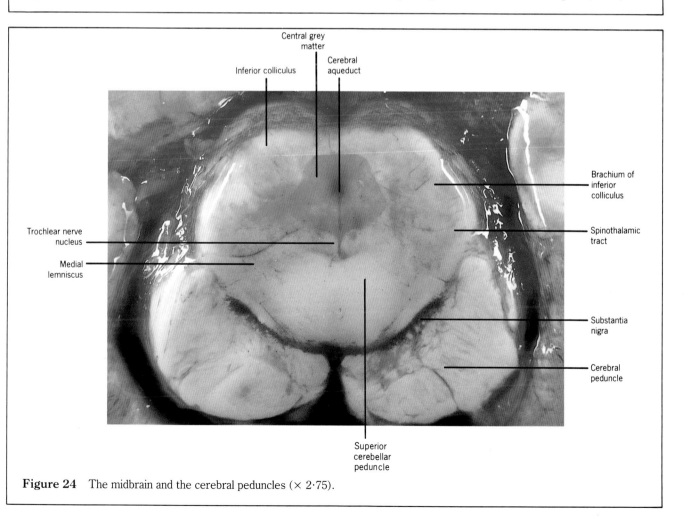

Central grey matter

Inferior colliculus

Cerebral aqueduct

Brachium of inferior colliculus

Spinothalamic tract

Trochlear nerve nucleus

Medial lemniscus

Substantia nigra

Cerebral peduncle

Superior cerebellar peduncle

Figure 24 The midbrain and the cerebral peduncles (× 2·75).

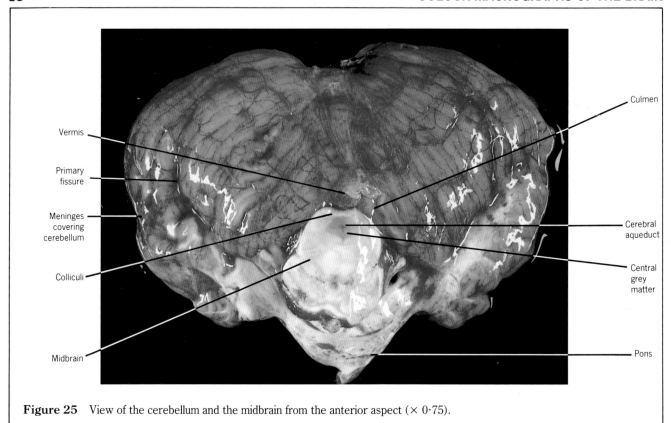

Figure 25   View of the cerebellum and the midbrain from the anterior aspect (× 0·75).

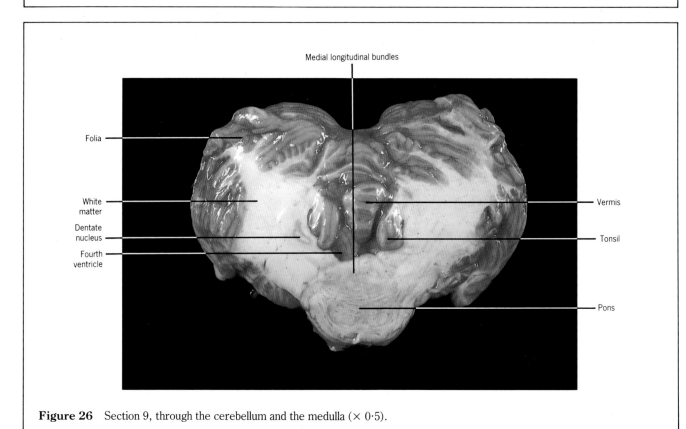

Figure 26   Section 9, through the cerebellum and the medulla (× 0·5).

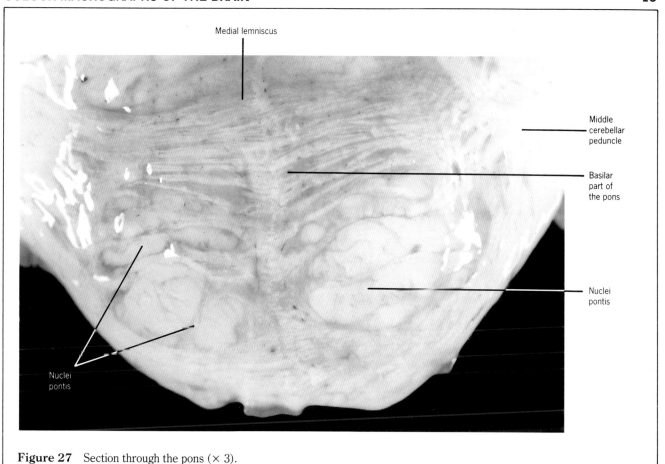

Figure 27   Section through the pons (× 3).

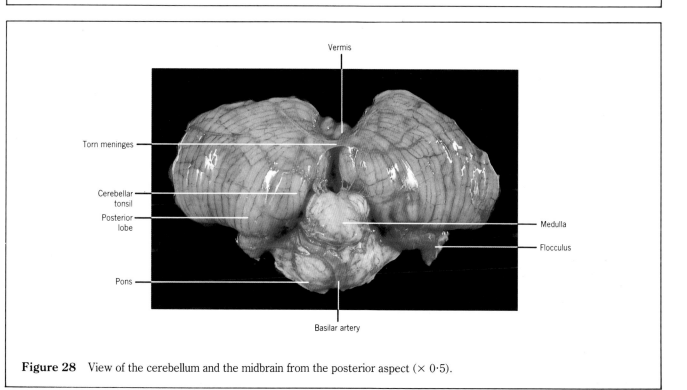

Figure 28   View of the cerebellum and the midbrain from the posterior aspect (× 0·5).

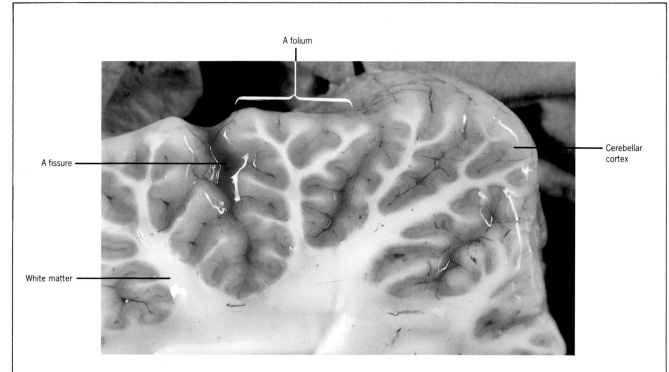

Figure 29   The arbor vitae appearance of a folium of the cerebellum (× 10).

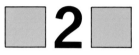

SECTION 2

MICROSCOPIC CONSTITUENT ELEMENTS

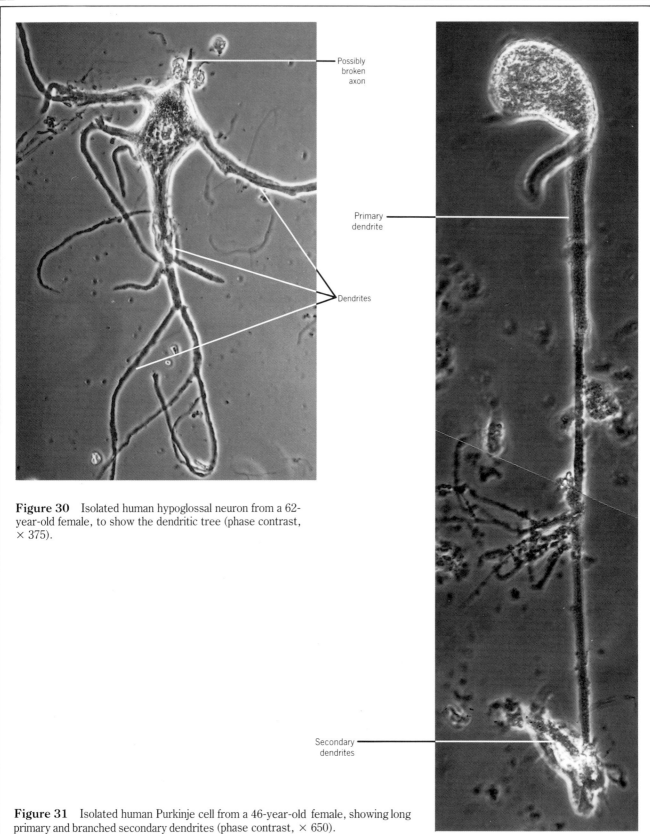

Figure 30   Isolated human hypoglossal neuron from a 62-year-old female, to show the dendritic tree (phase contrast, × 375).

Figure 31   Isolated human Purkinje cell from a 46-year-old female, showing long primary and branched secondary dendrites (phase contrast, × 650).

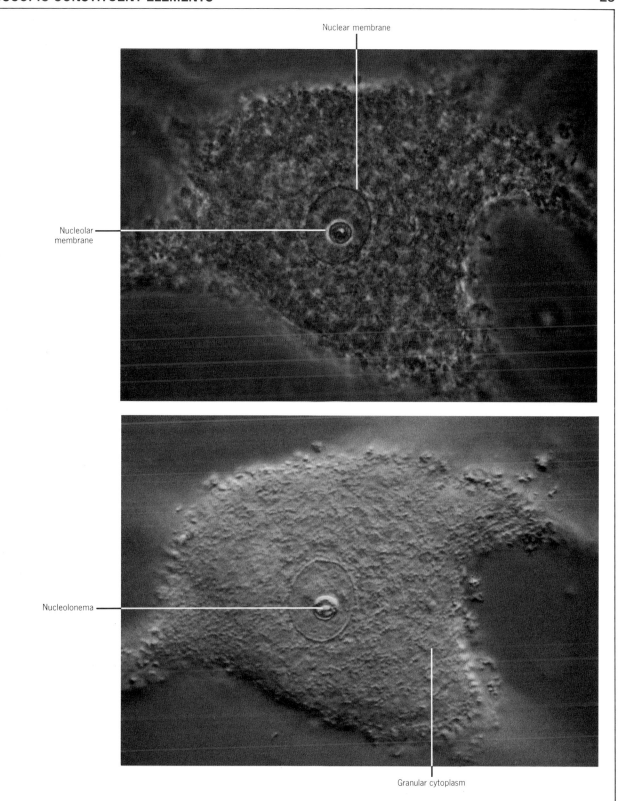

Figure 32 Isolated rabbit neuron from the lateral vestibular nucleus to show nuclear and nucleolar membranes, by phase contrast (above) and by differential interference contrast microscopy (below) (× 750). (These photographs were kindly taken by Mr M. I. Walker, of Stafford, using flash illumination.)

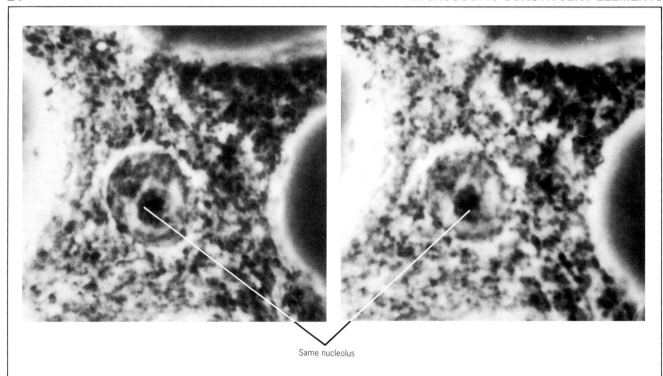

Same nucleolus

Figure 33 Isolated rabbit lateral vestibular neuron photographed twice with an interval of 20 minutes, to show nucleolar and cytoplasmic movements (phase contrast, × 2000).

Nucleolar membrane

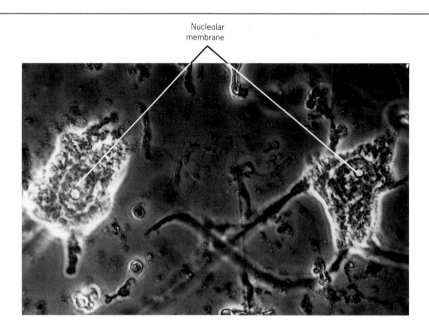

Figure 34 Isolated human neurons from the arcuate nucleus of a 71-year-old male, to show the nucleolar membranes (phase contrast, × 800).

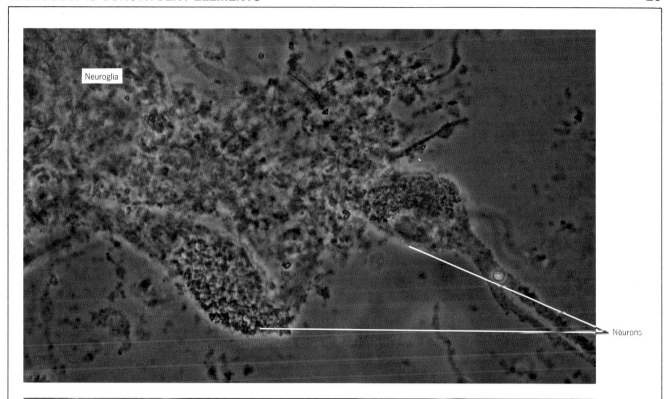

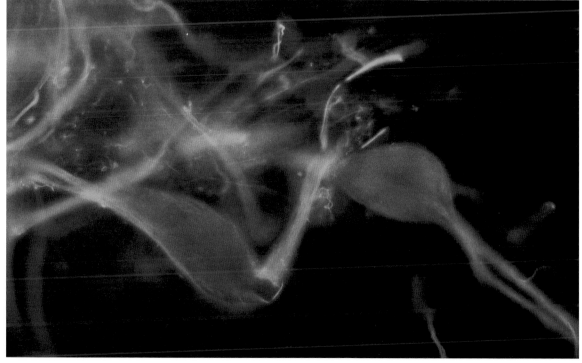

Figure 35 Teased human substantia nigral neurons and neuroglia from an 82-year-old male, by phase contrast (above) and stained with anti-neurofilament antibody (below) (× 500).

Note the fluorescence throughout the neuron, but not of the fine granular material.

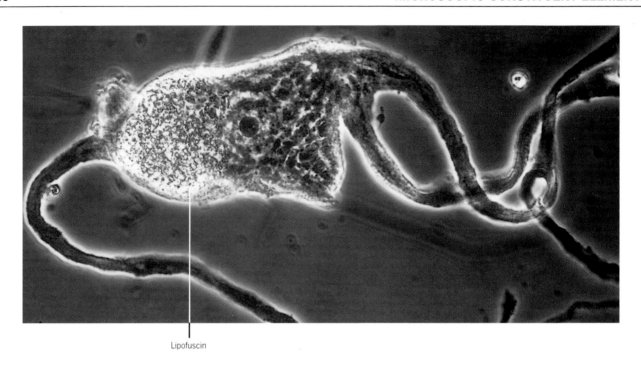

Lipofuscin

Figure 36   Isolated human ventral horn cell from the cervical spinal cord of a 75-year-old male, to show intracellular lipofuscin (phase contrast, × 800).

Lipofuscin accumulates with age.

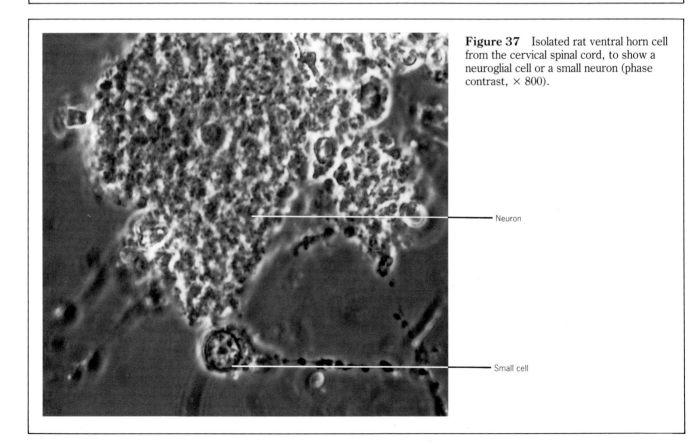

Figure 37   Isolated rat ventral horn cell from the cervical spinal cord, to show a neuroglial cell or a small neuron (phase contrast, × 800).

Neuron

Small cell

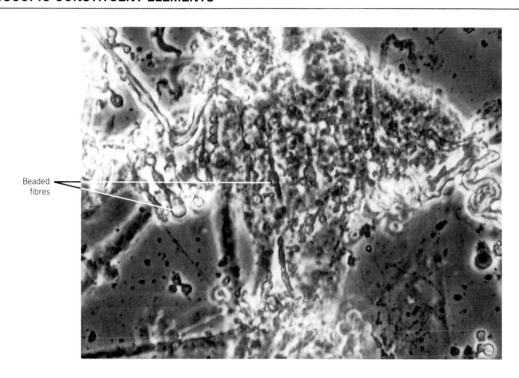

Beaded
fibres

Figure 38 Isolated rabbit ventral horn cell from the cervical spinal cord focused on the somal surface to show adherent beaded fibres (phase contrast, × 650).

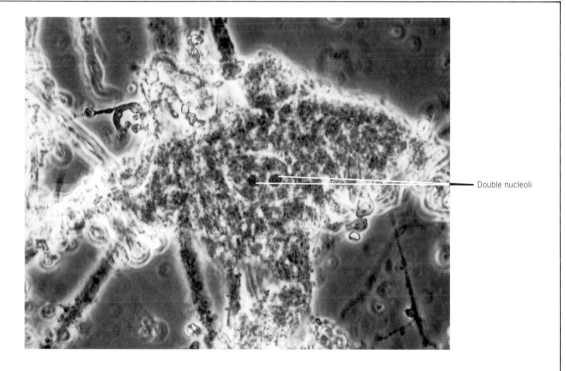

Double nucleoli

Figure 39 The same neuron as in the previous figure, but focused inside the cell to show the nucleus and paired nucleoli (phase contrast, × 650).

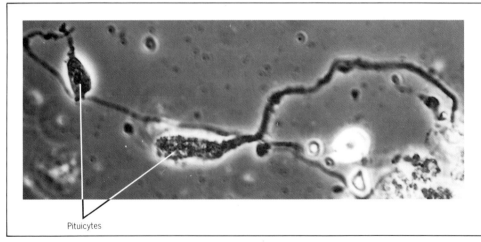

Figure 40 Isolated human pituicytes from a 54-year-old male (phase contrast, × 800).

Pituicytes

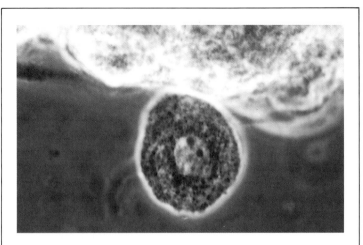

Figure 41 Isolated guinea-pig ganglion cell from the cervical spinal ganglion (phase contrast, × 800).

There are multiple nucleoli in this and the next figure.

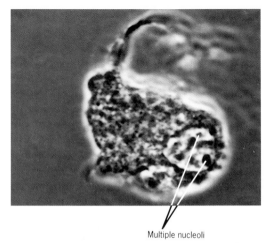

Multiple nucleoli

Figure 42 Isolated guinea-pig ganglion cell from the myenteric plexus of the colon (phase contrast, × 1300).

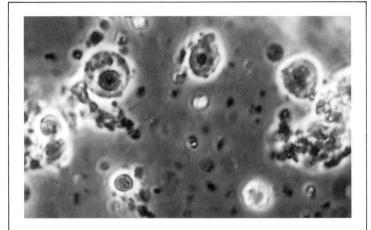

Figure 43 Isolated human neurons or neuroglial cells from the red nucleus of a 77-year-old male (phase contrast, × 800).

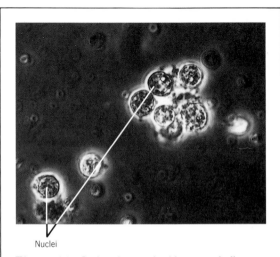

Nuclei

Figure 44 Isolated 1-week-old rat cerebellar granule cells (phase contrast, × 800).

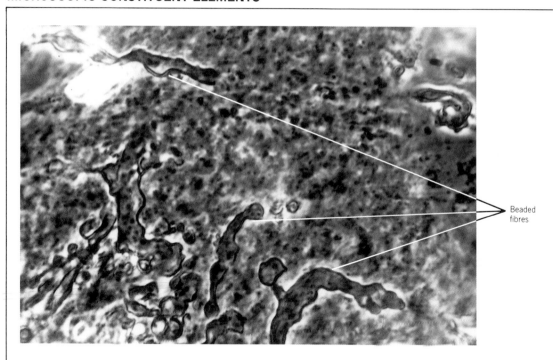

Figure 45 Surface of the soma of an isolated rabbit ventral horn cell from the cervical spinal cord to show adherent beaded fibre endings (phase contrast, × 1500).

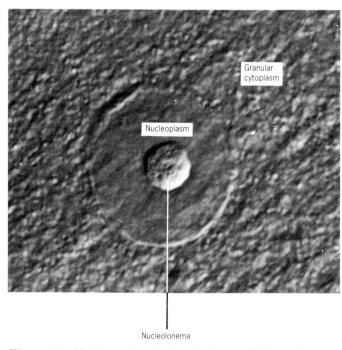

Figure 46 Nucleus and nucleolus of isolated rabbit lateral vestibular neuron (oblique negative phase contrast, × 1500). (By kind permission of Mr L. V. Martin, OBE.)

Note the granularity of the cytoplasm and the transparency of the nucleoplasm.

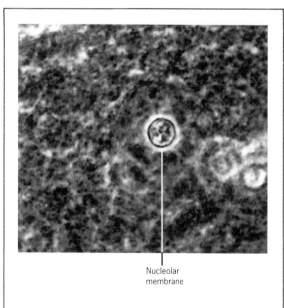

Figure 47 Nucleolar membrane and nucleolonema in isolated rabbit lateral vestibular neuron (phase contrast, × 1200).

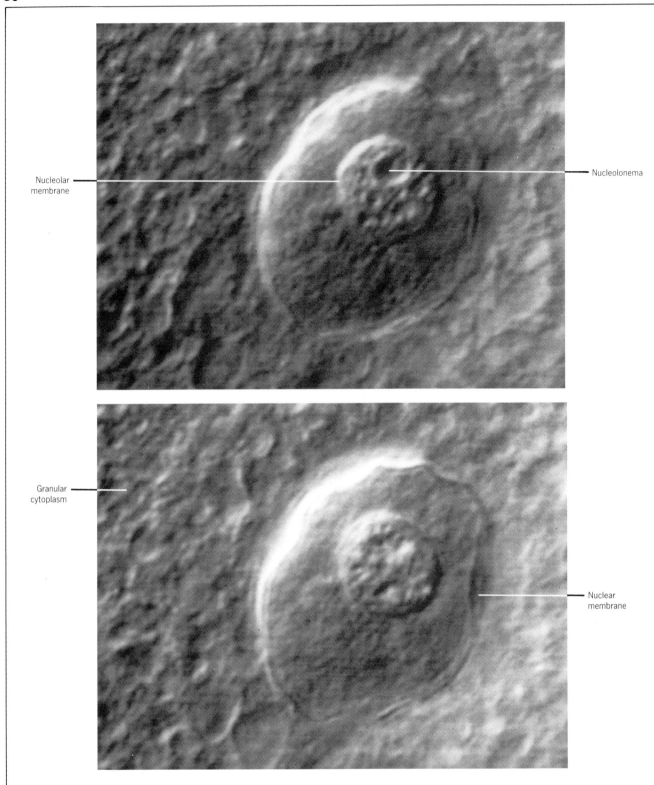

Nucleolar membrane

Nucleolonema

Granular cytoplasm

Nuclear membrane

Figures 48 and 49   Nucleus and nucleolus of isolated rabbit ventral horn cell to show the mitochondria and nucleolonema. These two optical sections were 1 μm apart (Zeiss scanning differential interference contrast, × 4300). (All differential interference micrographs were taken by kind permission of Miss P. Gunter of Zeiss Oberkochen.)

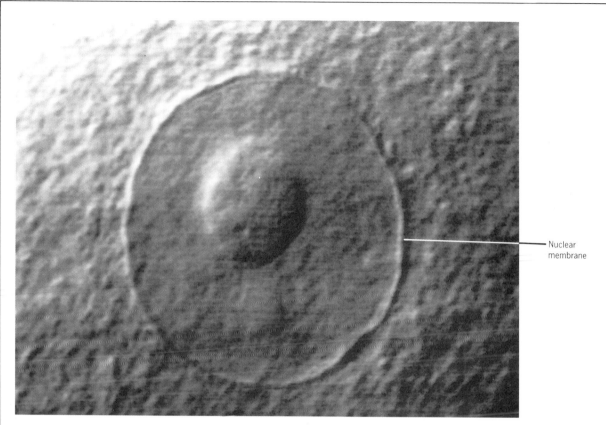

Figure 50 Nucleus and nucleolus of isolated rabbit lateral vestibular neuron to show the nuclear membrane (microscopy as in previous figure, × 4300).

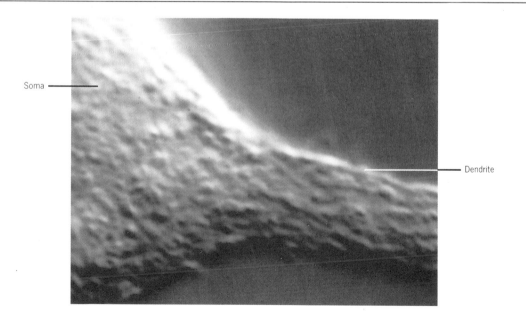

Figure 51 Soma–dendritic junction of isolated rabbit lateral vestibular neuron to show granular appearance (Zeiss scanning differential interference contrast, × 4300).

Granules

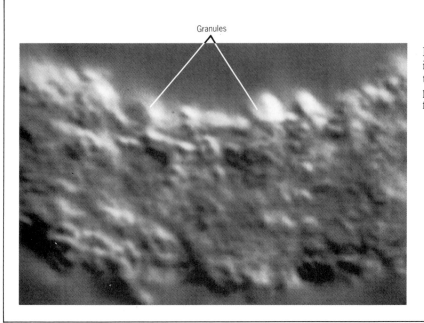

Figure 52   Surface of the dendrite of an isolated rabbit ventral horn neuron to show the granular appearance compared with the previous figure (microscopy as in previous figure, × 6800).

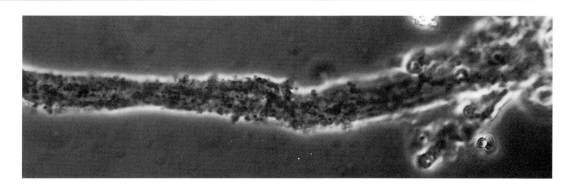

Figure 53   Isolated human dendrite from a Betz cell from a 55-year-old male, to show the dendritic structure and adherent fine granules (phase contrast, × 800).

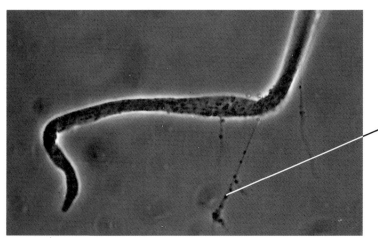

Figure 54   Isolated human dendrite from a vagal nucleus neuron of a 53-year-old male (phase contrast, × 800).

Note the fine adherent dendrites.

Fine dendrites

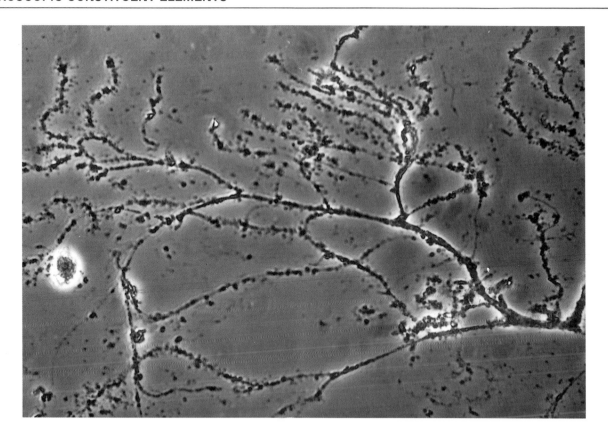

Figure 55 Isolated human dendritic tree of an inferior vestibular neuron from a 68-year-old male (phase contrast, × 750).

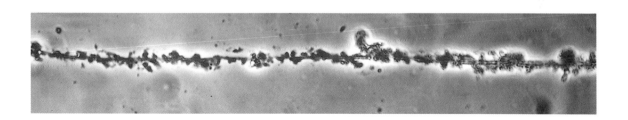

Figure 56 Isolated human fine fibre from the cerebellar grey matter from a 55-year-old male, to show adherent fine granules (phase contrast, × 750).

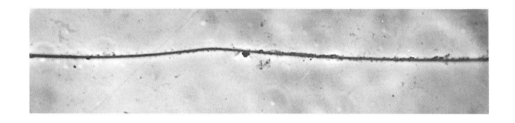

Figure 57 Isolated human fine fibre from the previous tissue, showing that it has a smooth outline (phase contrast, × 750).

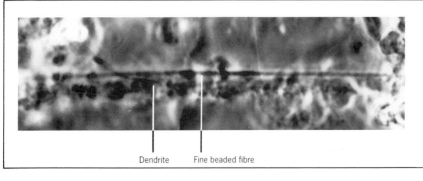

Dendrite   Fine beaded fibre

Figure 58 Isolated rabbit dendrite from a ventral horn cell from the cervical spinal cord, to show a fine beaded fibre running along its upper edge (phase contrast, × 2000).

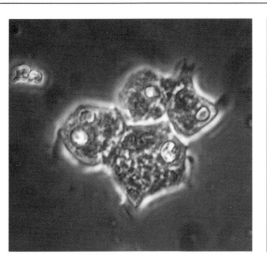 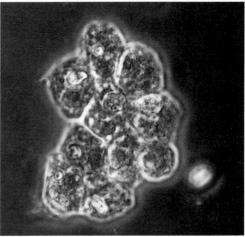

Figure 59 Isolated human ependymal cells from the wall of the lateral ventricle adjacent to the corpus callosum from a 68-year-old male (phase contrast, × 750).

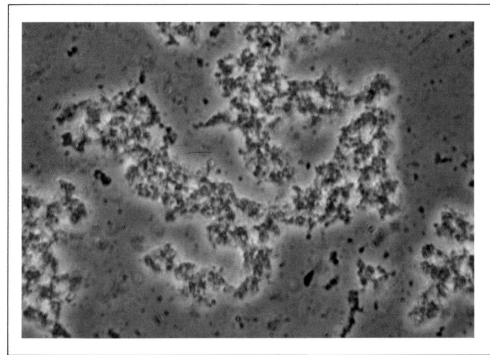

Figure 60 Teased human putamen from a 65-year-old female, to show fine granular material (phase contrast, × 750).

This material is the major component of neuroglia in grey matter.

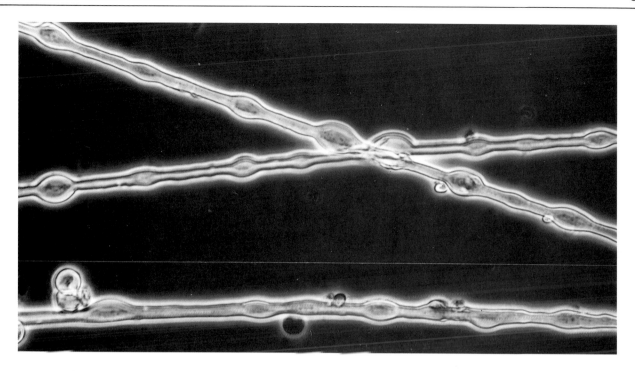

Figure 61 Isolated rat beaded fibres from dorsal white matter of cervical spinal cord to show small axoplasmic granules within the beads (phase contrast, × 800).

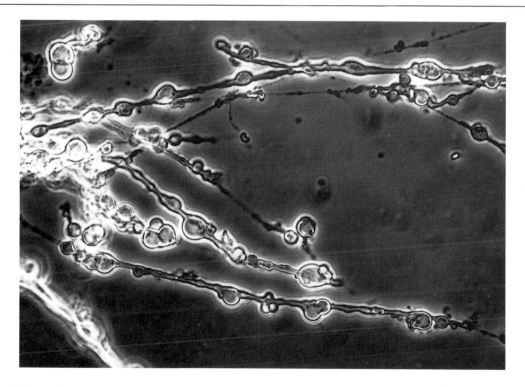

Figure 62 Teased human beaded fibres from the vestibulospinal tract of an 89-year-old female (phase contrast, × 800). The beads are refractile.

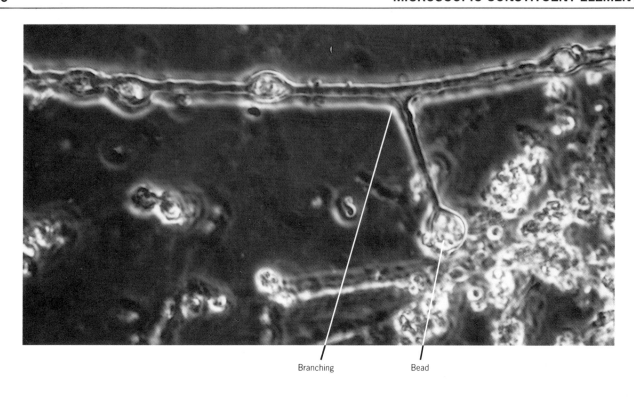

Branching   Bead

Figure 63   Isolated human beaded fibres from the pons of a 95-year-old female, to show a side branch ending in a bead (phase contrast, × 1300).

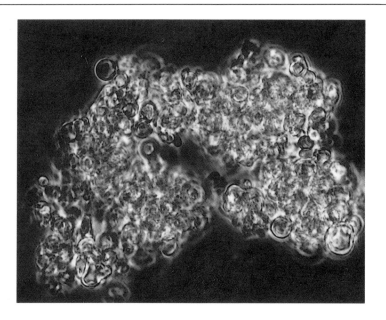

Figure 64   Clump of neuroglial droplets from the human cerebellar white matter of an 80-year-old female (phase contrast, × 800).

Droplets are a major component of white matter.

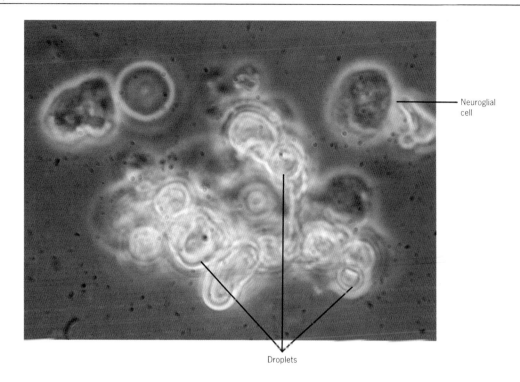

Neuroglial
cell

Droplets

Figure 65 Teased human optic nerve from a 43-year-old male, to show droplets and neuroglial cells (phase contrast, × 1500).

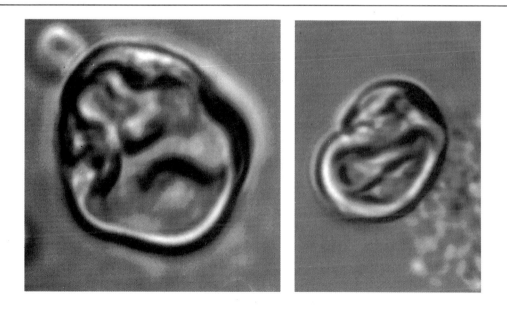

Figure 66 Isolated droplets from rabbit dorsal column of the spinal cord (Zeiss scanning differential interference contrast, × 4300).

These have not been seen before at high power.

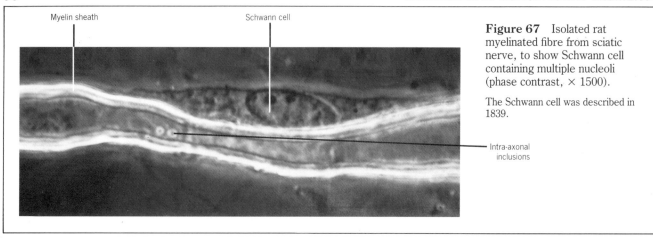

Figure 67   Isolated rat myelinated fibre from sciatic nerve, to show Schwann cell containing multiple nucleoli (phase contrast, × 1500).

The Schwann cell was described in 1839.

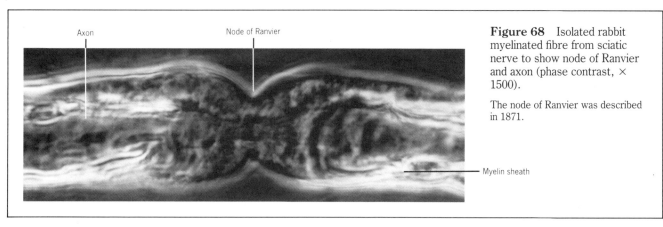

Figure 68   Isolated rabbit myelinated fibre from sciatic nerve to show node of Ranvier and axon (phase contrast, × 1500).

The node of Ranvier was described in 1871.

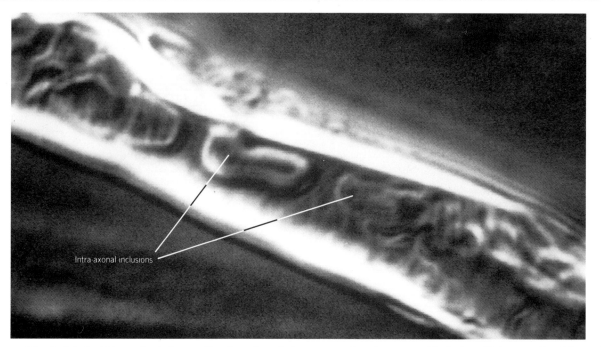

Figure 69   Isolated rabbit myelinated nerve fibre from the sciatic nerve, to show intra-axonal inclusions (Zeiss scanning differential interference contrast, × 4300).

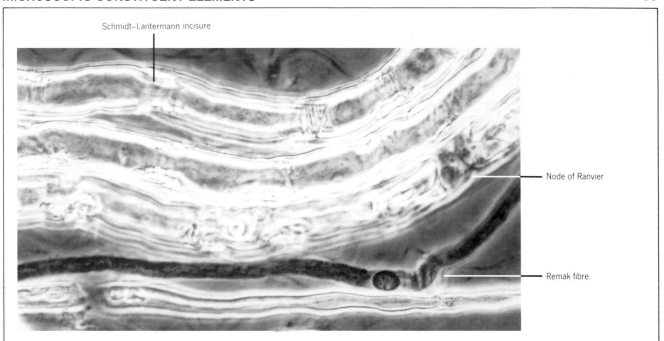

Schmidt–Lantermann incisure

Node of Ranvier

Remak fibre

Figure 70 Partially teased rabbit sciatic nerve showing a dark Remak fibre between myelinated fibres (phase contrast, × 750).

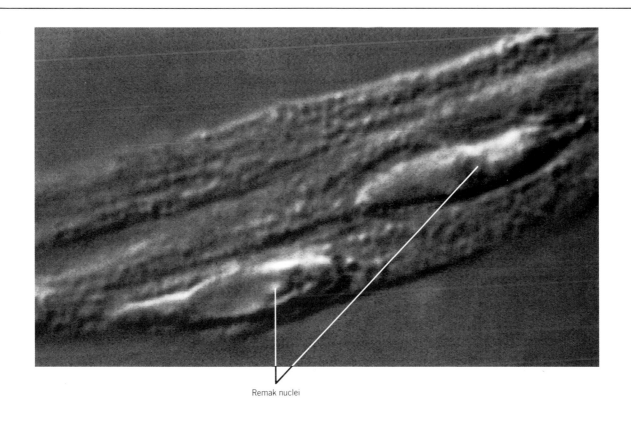

Remak nuclei

Figure 71 Isolated rabbit Remak fibres from the sciatic nerve (Zeiss scanning differential interference contrast, × 4000).

The elongated nuclei seen on the outside are characteristic of Remak (unmyelinated) fibres.

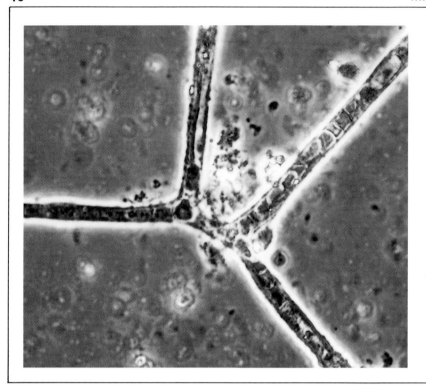

Figure 72 Isolated human capillary from the putamen of an 84-year-old male (phase contrast, × 750).

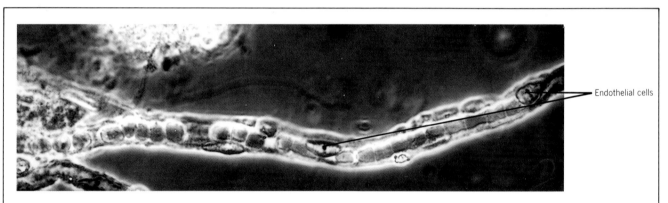

Endothelial cells

Figure 73 Isolated human capillary from the cerebellar cortex of a 55-year-old male, showing endothelial cells and/or pericytes (phase contrast, × 750).

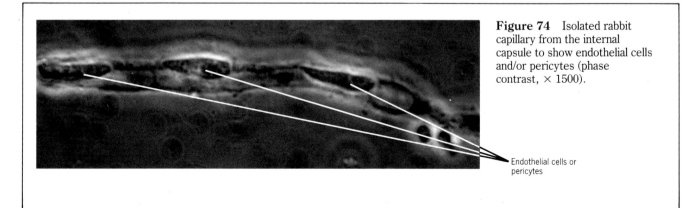

Figure 74 Isolated rabbit capillary from the internal capsule to show endothelial cells and/or pericytes (phase contrast, × 1500).

Endothelial cells or pericytes

SECTION 3

CEREBRAL CORTEX

Figure 75   Thin slab of adult rabbit frontal cortical grey matter, lightly coloured with methylene blue to show the incidence of neuron somas; **a–f** are successive, but not continuous from the surface of the cortex to the white matter. The laminae are indicated with Roman numerals: I, plexiform; II, external granular; III, pyramidal; IV, internal granular; V, ganglionic; VI, multiform (bright field, × 85).

The total thickness of the cortex in this specimen was 6 mm.

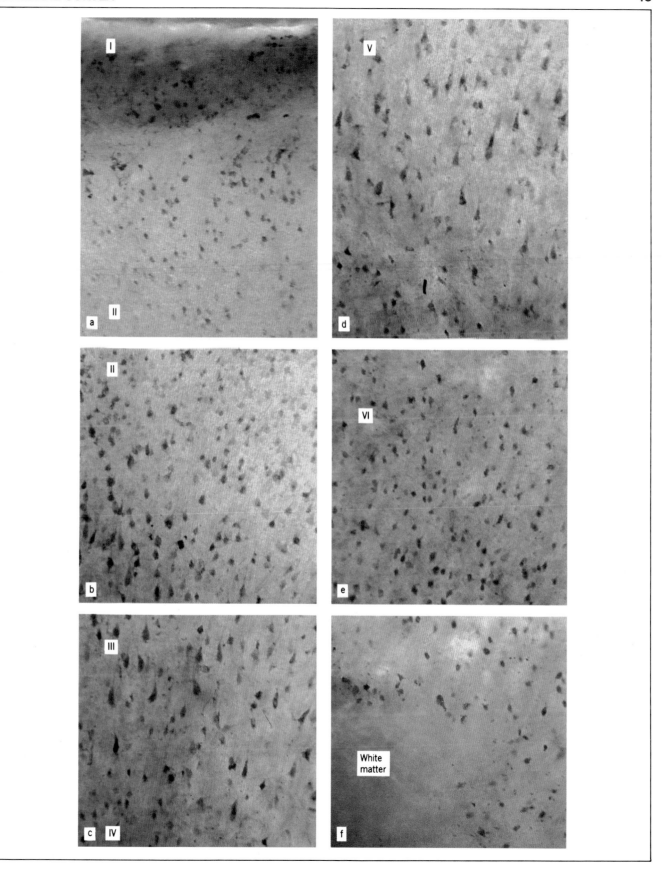

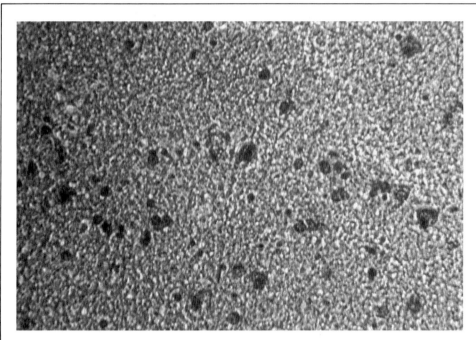

Figure 76   Thin slab of human frontal cortical grey matter from a 79-year-old male, lightly coloured with methylene blue to show the incidence of neuron somas (bright field, × 250).

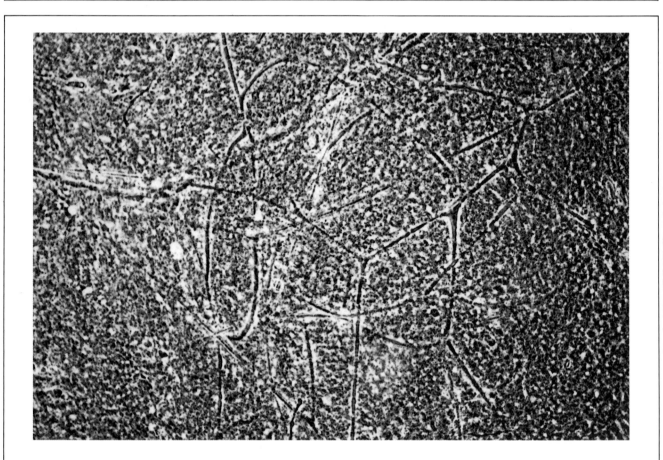

Figure 77   Thin slab of adult rat frontal cortical grey matter, unstained (phase contrast, × 335).

There is a rich blood supply, which gives part of the colour to grey matter.

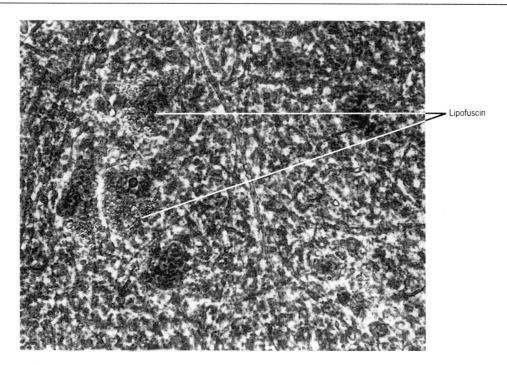

Figure 78 Thin slab of human frontal cortical grey matter from a 68-year-old male, to show neurons *in situ* (phase contrast, × 700).

Lipofuscin is present in the cytoplasm of most adult human neurons.

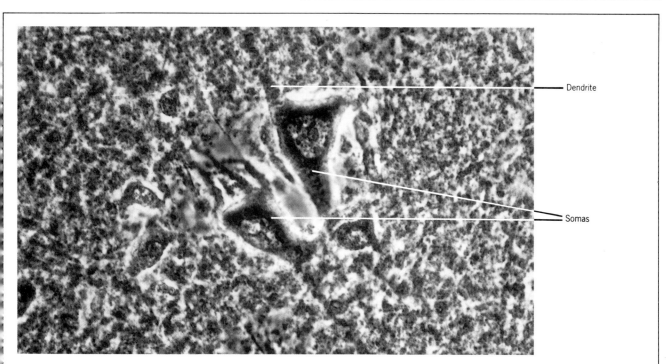

Figure 79 Thin slab of new-born lamb frontal cortical grey matter to show pyramidal neuronal somas *in situ* (phase contrast, × 700).

The dendrites are visible and the nucleus has a low refractive index.

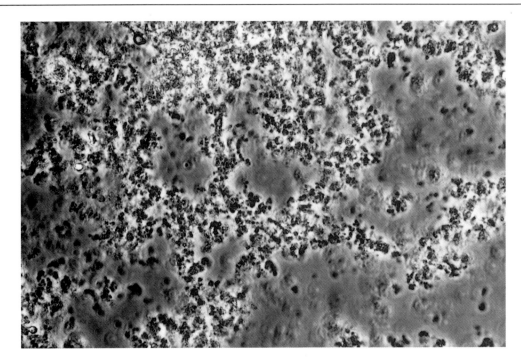

Figure 80   Teased fine granular material from human frontal grey matter from a 68-year-old male, to show individual or aggregates of granules (phase contrast, × 700).

These fine dark granules occupy most of the volume between the neurons in grey matter.

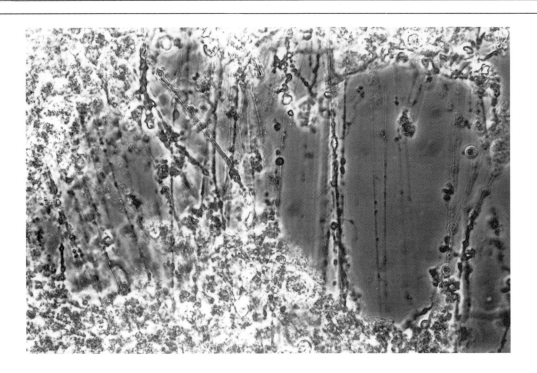

Figure 81   Teased human frontal grey matter from a 68-year-old male, to show fine fibres (phase contrast, × 700).

The fibres are seen clearly only when the tissue is teased, and fine granules often adhere to them.

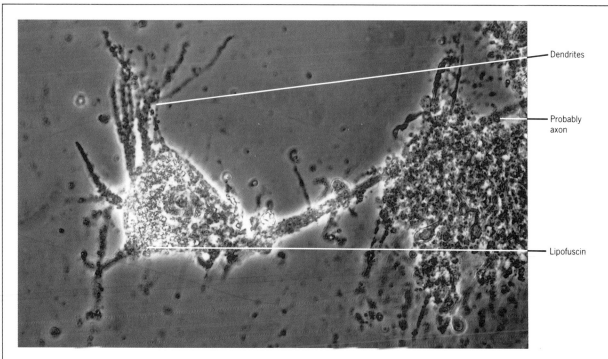

Figure 82 Teased human frontal grey matter from a 77-year-old male, to show a neuron and associated neuroglia (phase contrast, × 700).

Note the number of primary dendrites.

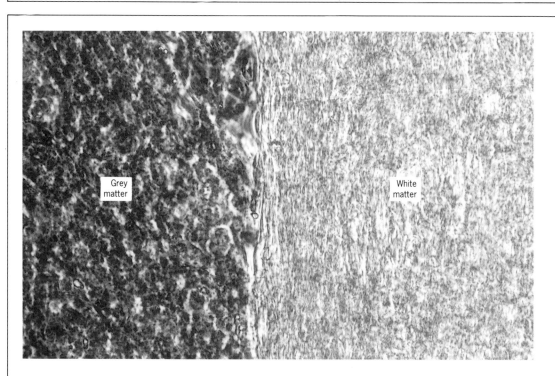

Figure 83 Thin slab of human frontal region from an 84-year-old male, to show grey–white matter boundary (phase contrast, × 700).

The grey matter has a high refractive index. There are fibres in the white matter.

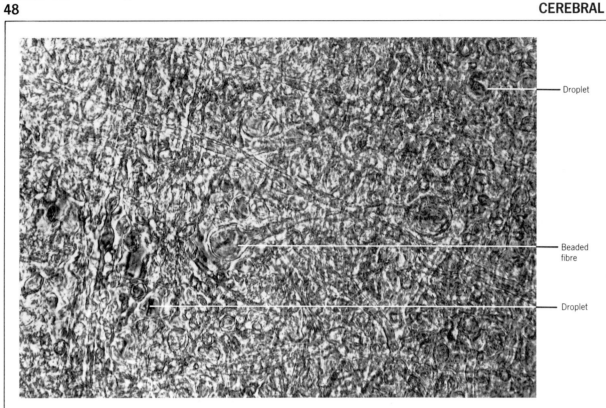

— Droplet

— Beaded
fibre

— Droplet

Figure 84   Thin slab of human frontal white matter from a 68-year-old male, to show beaded fibres and large droplets (phase contrast, × 700).

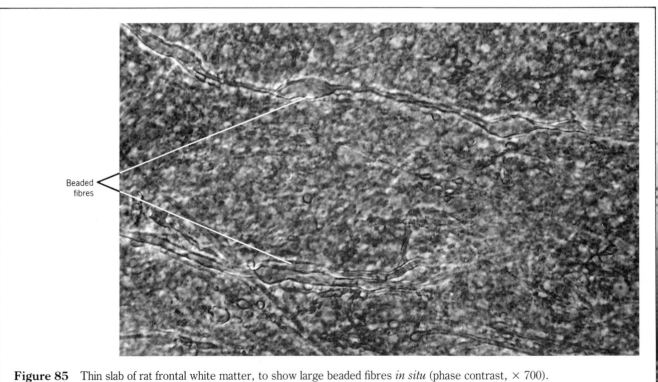

Beaded
fibres

Figure 85   Thin slab of rat frontal white matter, to show large beaded fibres *in situ* (phase contrast, × 700).

These droplets and beaded fibres were reported by Ehrenberg in 1833 and Remak in 1836, and more recently by Fernandez-Moran in 1952.

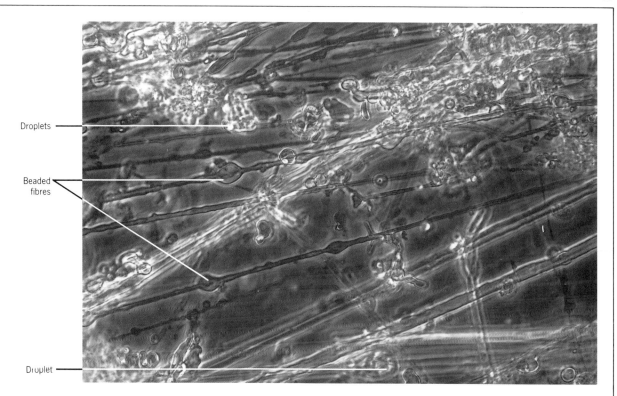

Droplets

Beaded
fibres

Droplet

Figure 86   Partially teased human frontal white matter of an 84-year-old male, to show beaded fibres and droplets (phase contrast, × 700).

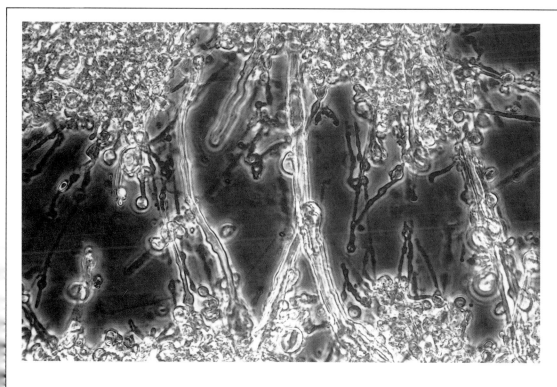

Figure 87   As previous figure, but from a 68-year-old male.

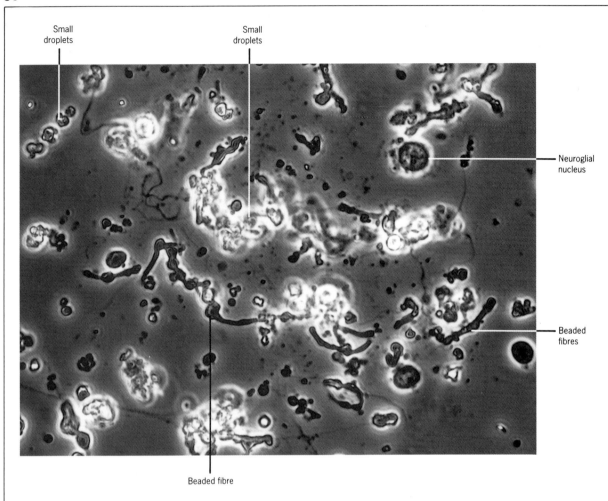

Small
droplets

Small
droplets

Neuroglial
nucleus

Beaded
fibres

Beaded fibre

Figure 88   Teased human frontal white matter from a 77-year-old male, to show fine beaded fibres and small droplets (phase contrast, × 800).

Neuroglial nuclei can be seen.

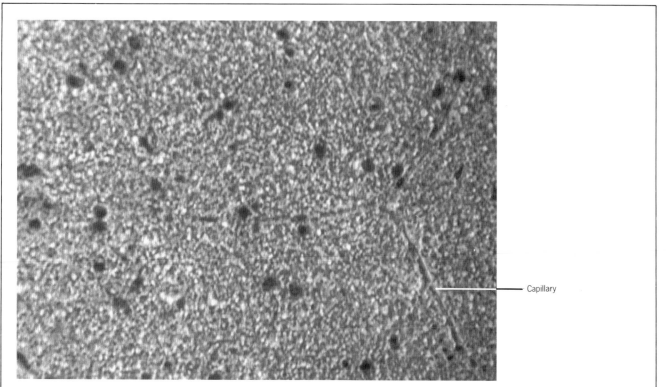

Capillary

Figure 89 Thin slab of human parietal cortical grey matter from a 79-year-old male, lightly coloured with methylene blue to show the incidence of neuron somas (bright field, × 300).

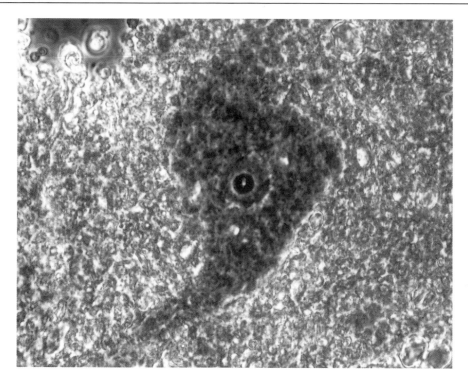

Figure 90 Thin slab of human parietal grey matter from a 53-year-old male, to show a Betz cell *in situ* (phase contrast, × 700).

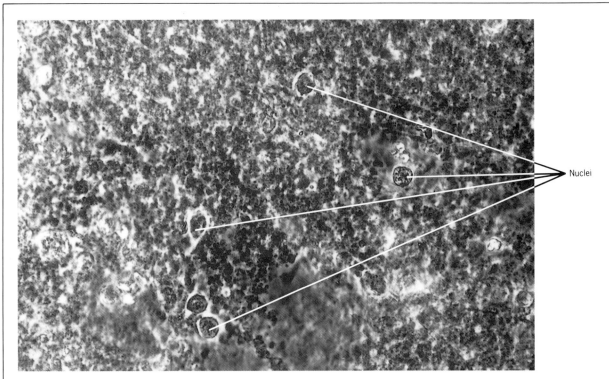

Figure 91 Thin slab of human parietal grey matter from a 68-year-old male to show neuroglial nuclei and fine granular material *in situ* (phase contrast, × 700).

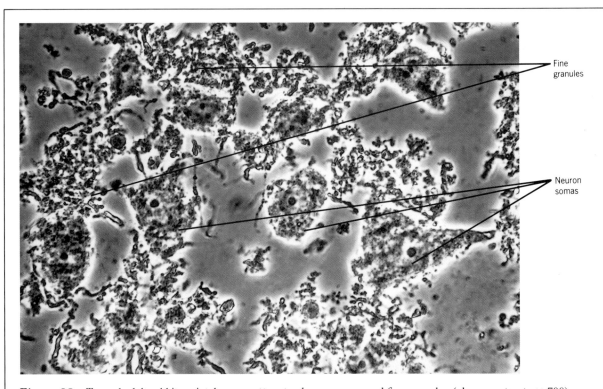

Figure 92 Teased adult rabbit parietal grey matter, to show neurons and fine granules (phase contrast, × 700).

The appearance of isolated neurons was first reported by Remak in 1838.

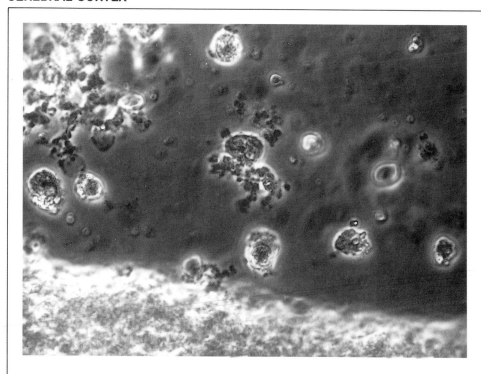

Figure 93 Teased human parietal grey matter from a 68-year-old male to show neuroglial nuclei or small neurons (phase contrast, × 700).

Note the absence of fibres attached to these cells. Neuroglial nuclei were first described by Virchow in 1856.

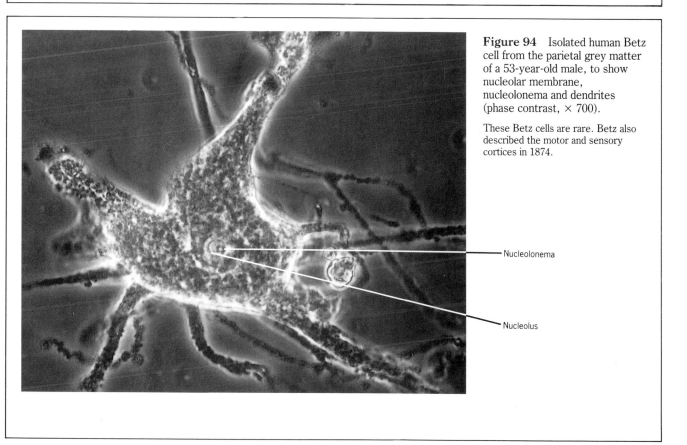

Figure 94 Isolated human Betz cell from the parietal grey matter of a 53-year-old male, to show nucleolar membrane, nucleolonema and dendrites (phase contrast, × 700).

These Betz cells are rare. Betz also described the motor and sensory cortices in 1874.

— Nucleolonema

— Nucleolus

Nucleolar
membrane

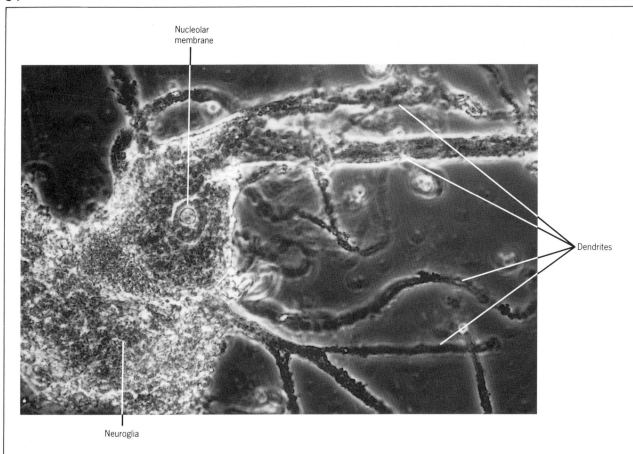

Dendrites

Neuroglia

Figure 95   Isolated human Betz cell from parietal grey matter of a 55-year-old male, to show intracellular lipofuscin, a nucleolar membrane and adherent neuroglia (phase contrast, × 700).

Lipofuscin was first seen in human brains by Obersteiner in 1903.

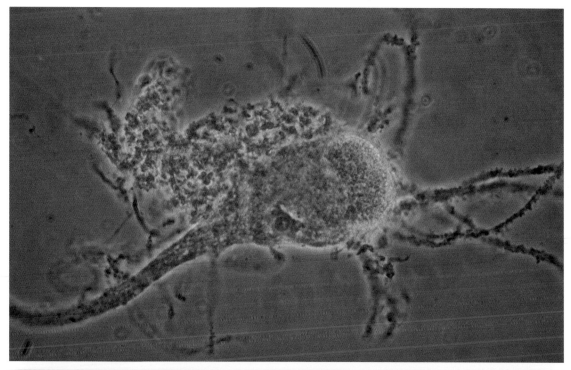

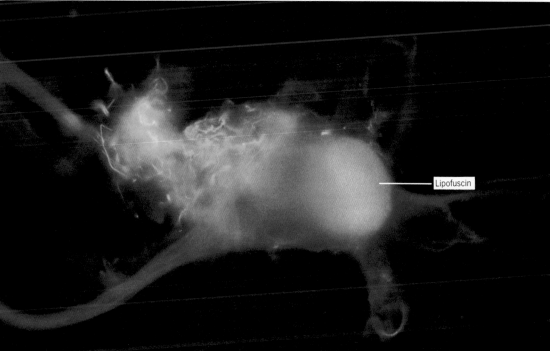

Lipofuscin

Figure 96 Isolated human Betz cell from an 82-year-old male, stained with anti-neurofilament 200 kD protein, by phase contrast (above) and after excitation with the blue light of 450–490 nm (below) (× 500).

The autofluorescence of lipofuscin is increased after antibody staining. There is little fluorescence in dendrites or fine granular material, but some fine fibres in the neuroglia fluoresce intensely.

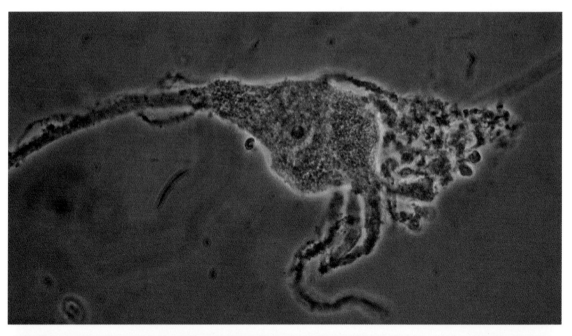

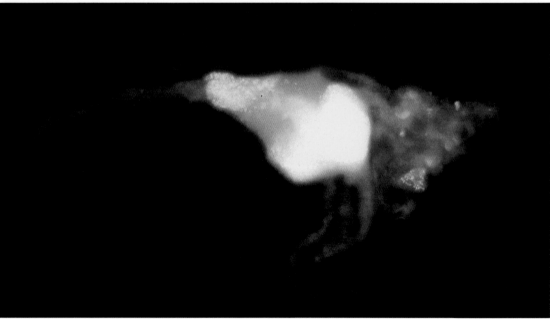

Figure 97 Isolated human Betz cell from an 82-year-old male, stained with anti-glial fibrillary acidic protein, by phase contrast (above) and after excitation with blue light of 450–490 nm (below) (× 500).

Neither the dendrites nor the neuroglial fibres fluoresce. Compare with Figure 96.

Figure 98 Isolated clump of fine granular material from human parietal cortex of a 68-year-old male, and a neuroglial nucleus or small cell below it (phase contrast, × 800).

This material is a major component of the neuroglia between neurons. Neuroglia was first described by Virchow in 1846.

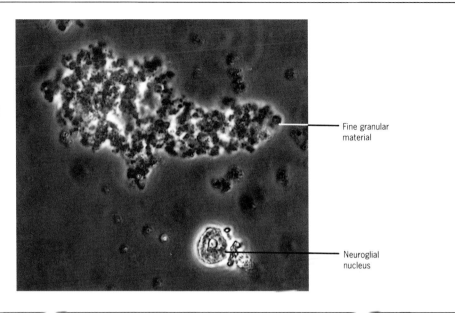

Fine granular material

Neuroglial nucleus

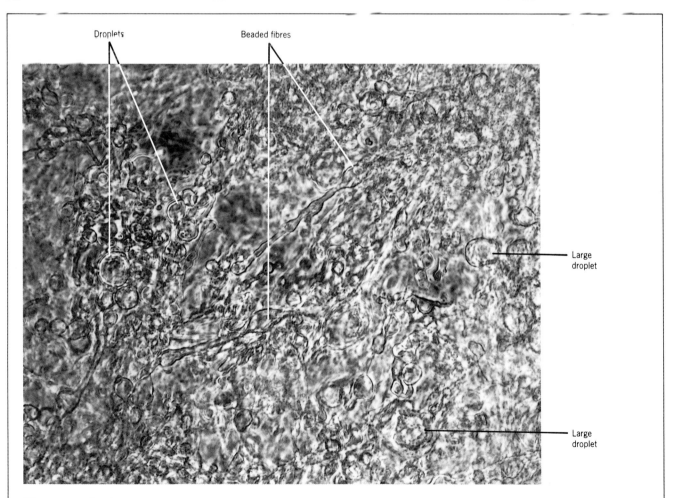

Droplets

Beaded fibres

Large droplet

Large droplet

Figure 99 Partially teased thin slab of human parietal white matter from a 68-year-old male, to show beaded fibres and large droplets (phase contrast, × 800).

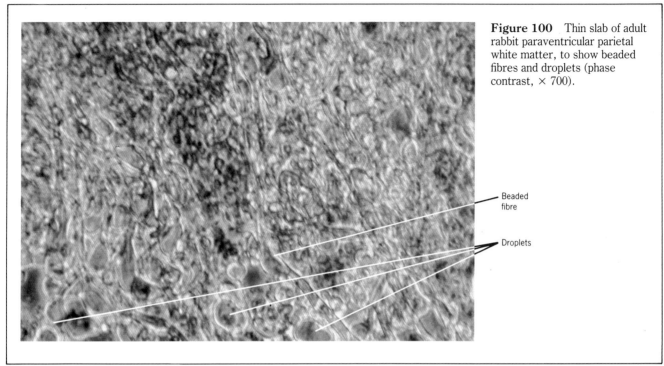

Figure 100   Thin slab of adult rabbit paraventricular parietal white matter, to show beaded fibres and droplets (phase contrast, × 700).

Beaded fibre

Droplets

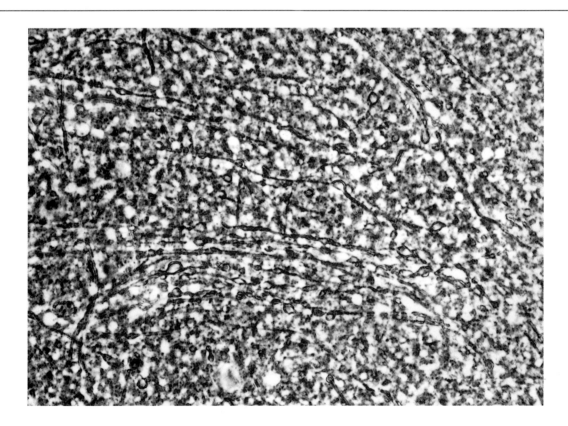

Figure 101   Thin slab of guinea-pig parietal white matter to show fibres (phase contrast, ×700).

White matter was first described by de Vieussens in 1684.

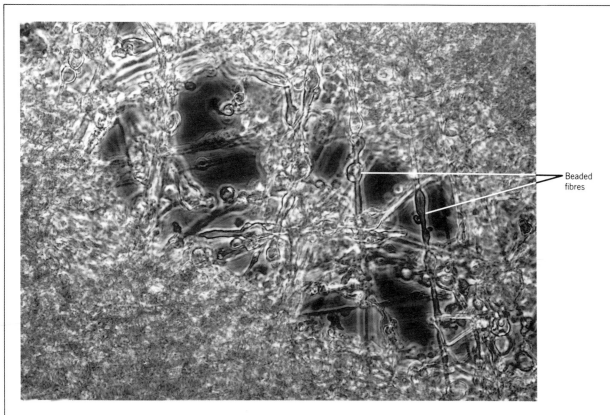

Beaded
fibres

Figure 102 Partially teased thin slab of human parietal white matter from a 68-year-old male, to show beaded fibres travelling in several directions (phase contrast, × 700).

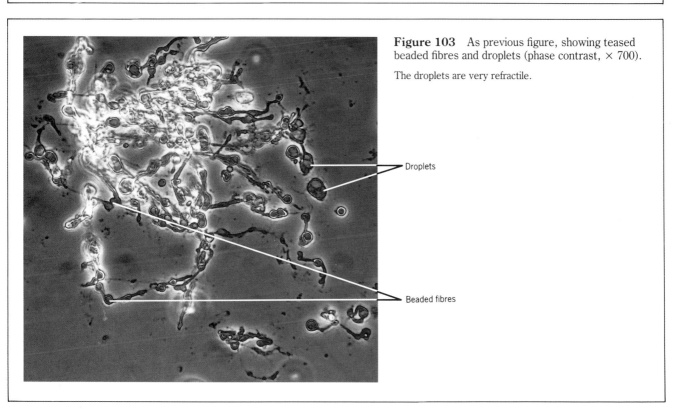

Figure 103 As previous figure, showing teased beaded fibres and droplets (phase contrast, × 700).

The droplets are very refractile.

Droplets

Beaded fibres

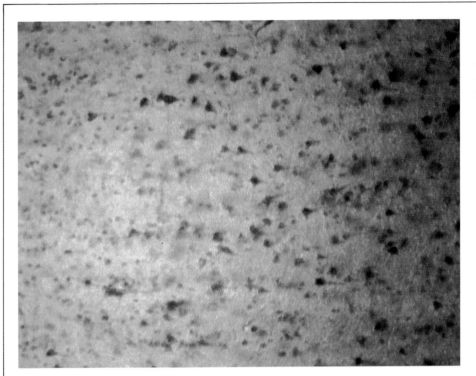

Figure 104 Thin slab of human temporal grey matter from a 79-year-old male, lightly coloured with methylene blue to show the incidence of neuron somas (bright field, × 110).

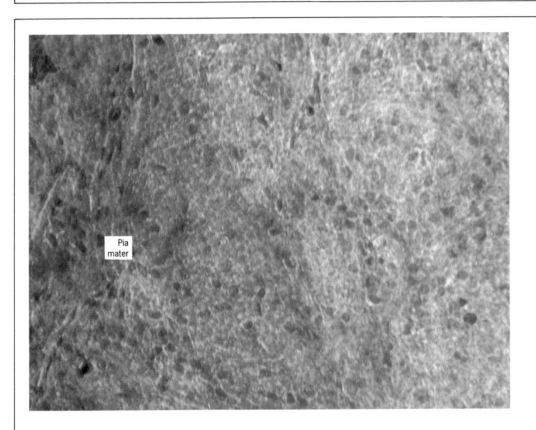

Figure 105 Thin slab of human temporal cortex from a 79-year-old male, lightly coloured with methylene blue, covered by the pia mater on the left (bright field, × 255).

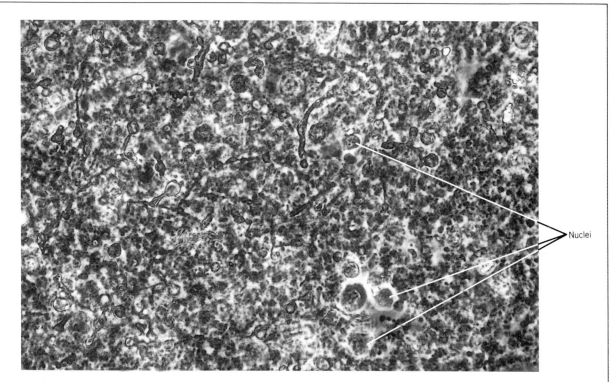

Nuclei

Figure 106   Thin slab of human temporal grey matter from a 73-year-old male, to show neuronal somas and beaded fibres (phase contrast, × 700).

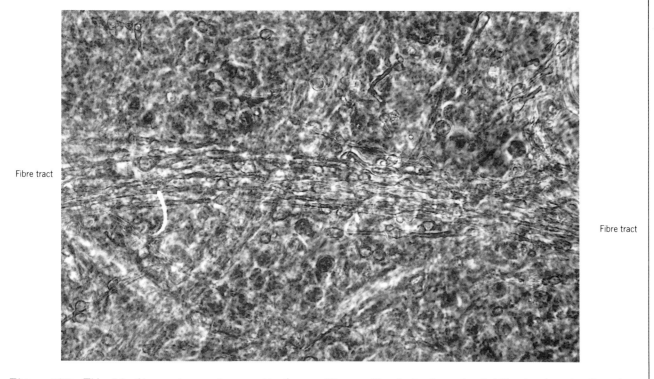

Fibre tract

Fibre tract

Figure 107   Thin slab of human temporal grey matter from an 84-year-old male, to show a beaded fibre tract passing through (phase contrast, × 700).

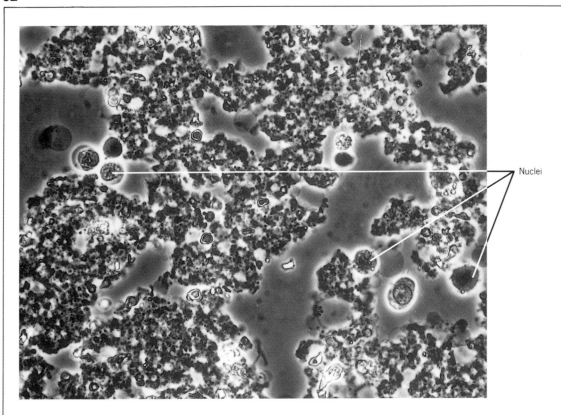

Nuclei

Figure 108   Teased human temporal grey matter of an 84-year-old male, to show cells with large nuclei and fine granular material (phase contrast, × 700).

Figure 109   Teased human temporal grey matter from a 73-year-old male, to show small neurons or neuroglial nuclei and fine granular material (phase contrast, × 700).

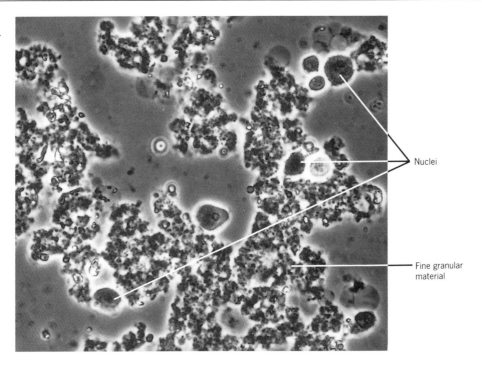

Nuclei

Fine granular material

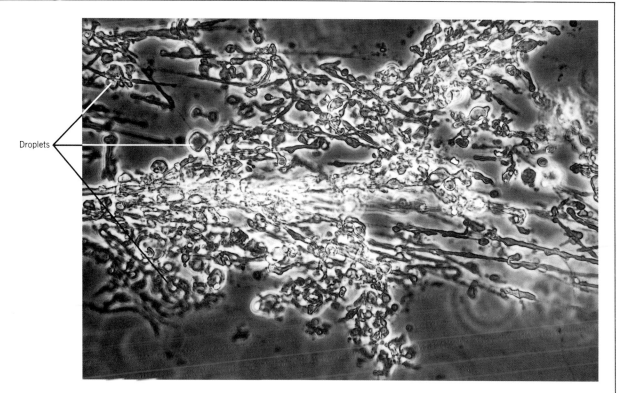

Figure 110 Teased human temporal white matter from an 84-year-old male, to show beaded fibres and droplets (phase contrast, × 700).

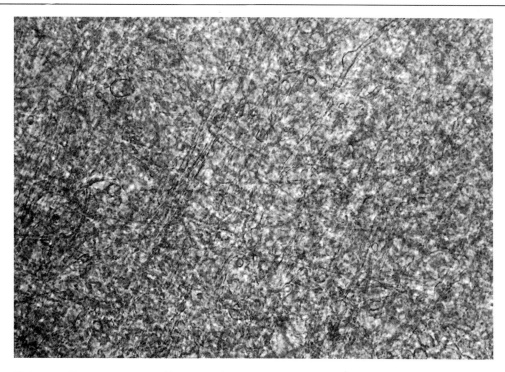

Figure 111 Thin slab of human temporal white matter from an 84-year-old male, to show small beaded fibres (phase contrast, × 640).

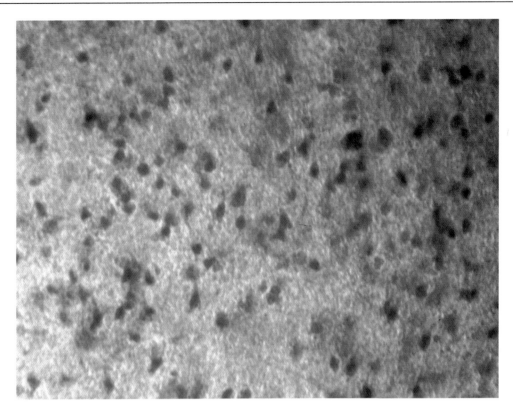

Figure 112 Thin slab of human occipital grey matter from a 79-year-old male, lightly coloured with methylene blue to show the incidence of neuron somas (bright field, × 300).

Figure 113 Thin slab of human occipital grey–white matter boundary from a 79-year-old male, lightly coloured with methylene blue (bright field, × 300).

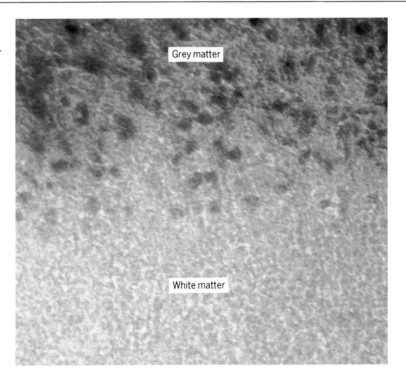

Grey matter

White matter

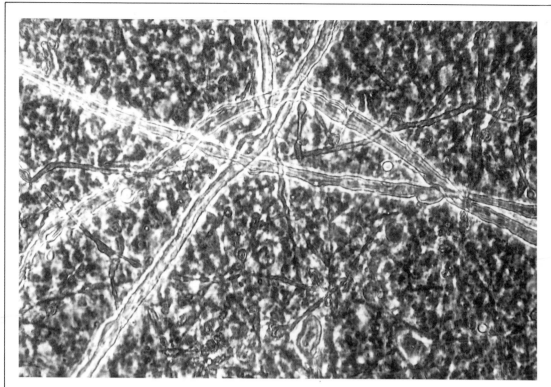

Figure 114   Thin slab of human occipital grey matter from a 68-year-old male, to show large beaded fibres (phase contrast, × 700).

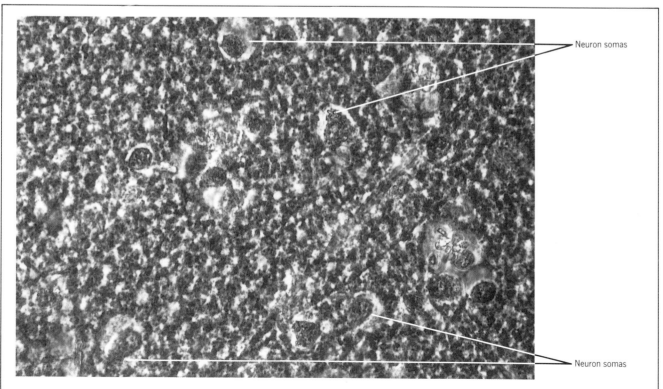

Figure 115   Thin slab of human occipital grey matter from a 68-year old male, to show neurons *in situ* (phase contrast, × 700).

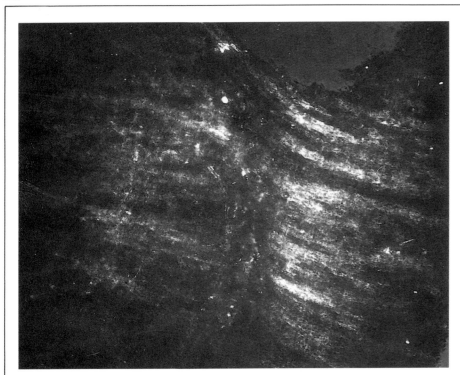

Figure 116   Thin slab of human occipital grey matter from a 55-year-old male, to show birefringence of fibres (polarized light, × 130).

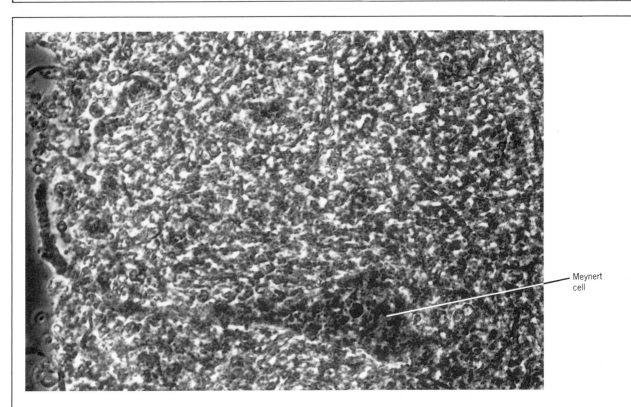

Meynert cell

Figure 117   Thin slab of human occipital grey matter from a 73-year-old male, to show a Meynert cell *in situ* (phase contrast, × 700).

There are few of these cells. They were first seen by Meynert in 1872.

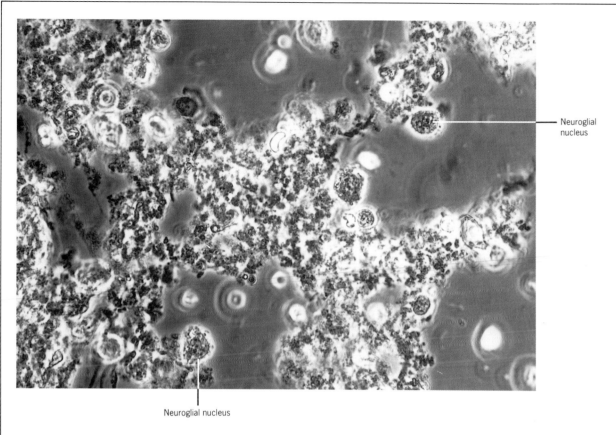

Figure 118 Teased human occipital grey matter from a 68-year-old male, to show neuroglial nuclei and fine granular material (phase contrast, × 700).

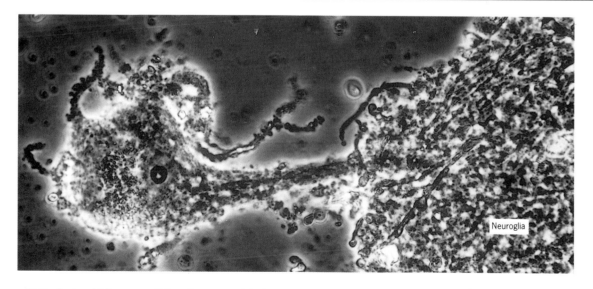

Figure 119 Isolated Meynert cell from human occipital grey matter from a 77-year-old male (phase contrast, × 800).

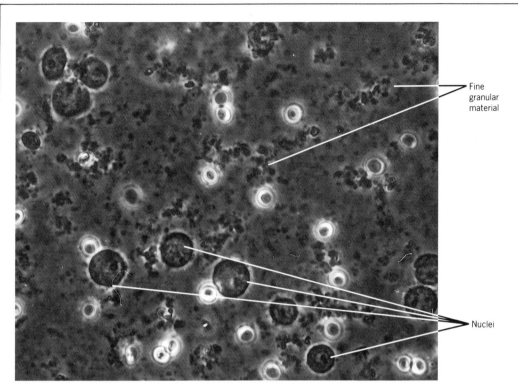

Figure 120   Teased rat occipital grey matter to show neuroglial nuclei or cells (phase contrast, × 700).

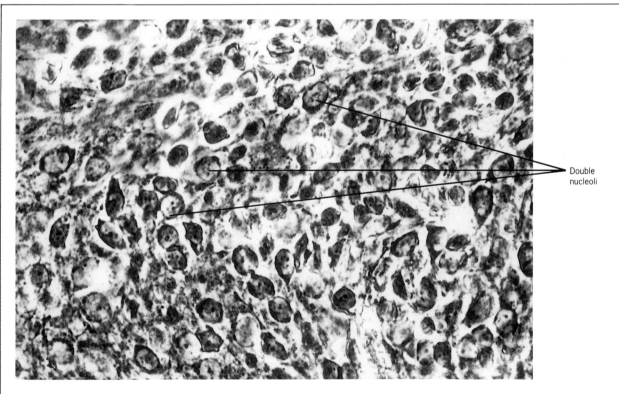

Figure 121   Thin slab of new-born mouse occipital grey matter, to show neurons — some with double nucleoli (phase contrast, × 700).

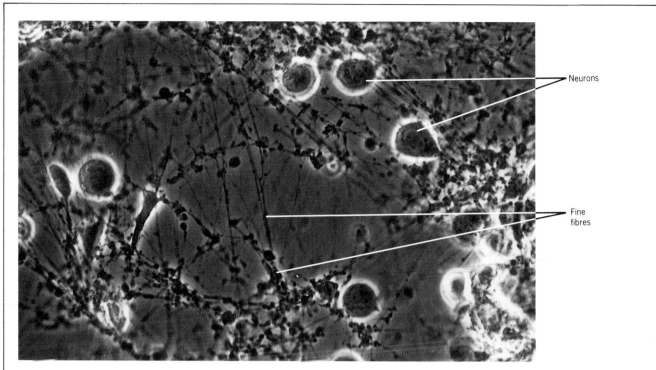

Figure 122 Teased new-born mouse occipital grey matter, to show neurons with little cytoplasm and fine fibres (phase contrast, × 700).

Fine fibres can be seen only in the teased tissue.

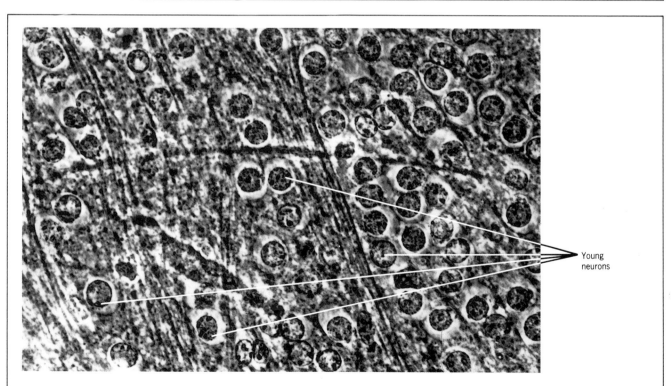

Figure 123 Thin slab of new-born mouse occipital white matter, to show probable migration of cells (phase contrast, × 700).

The cytoplasm of the neurons is transparent at this age.

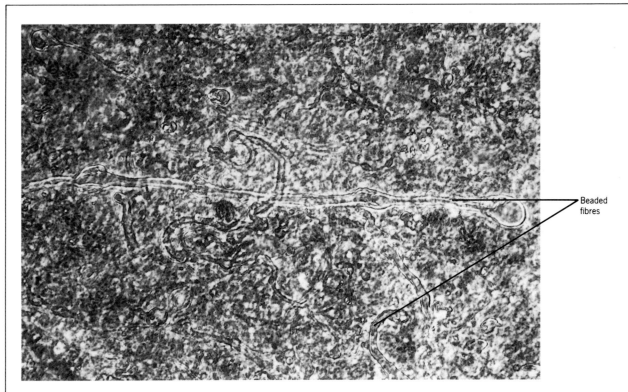

Figure 124 Thin slab of human occipital white matter from a 68-year-old male, to show beaded fibres (phase contrast, × 700).

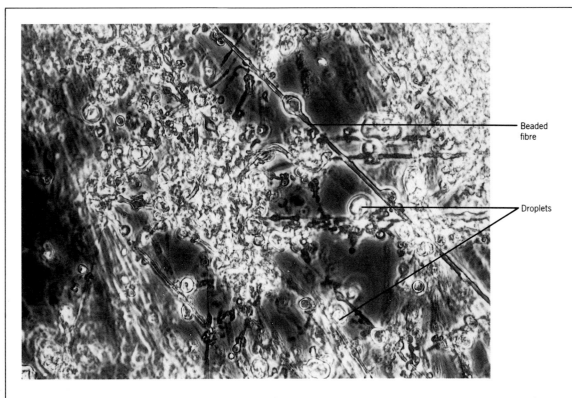

Figure 125 As previous figure, to show teased beaded fibres and large droplets (phase contrast, × 700).

SECTION
4

SUBCORTICAL STRUCTURES

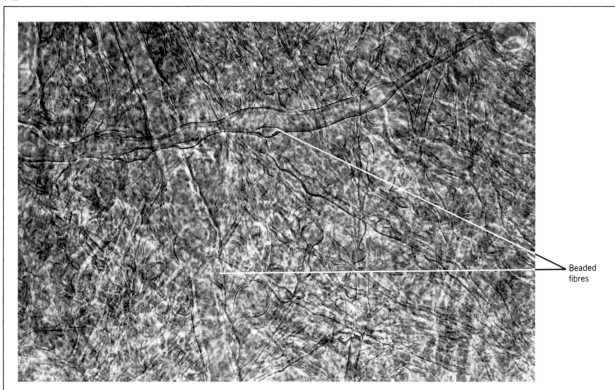

Figure 126   Thin slab of human corpus callosum from an 82-year-old female, to show beaded fibres (phase contrast, × 700).

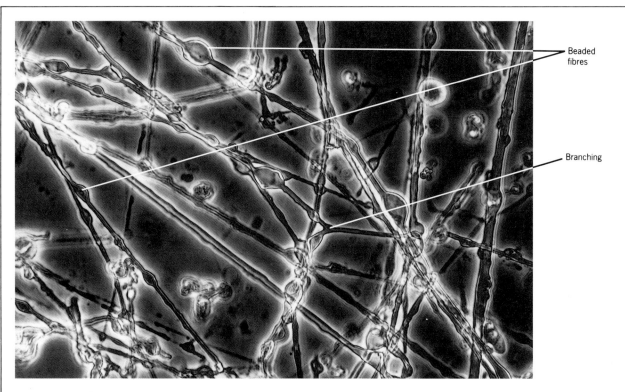

Figure 127   Teased human corpus callosum from a 77-year-old male, to show beaded fibres, which can occasionally be seen branching (phase contrast, × 700).

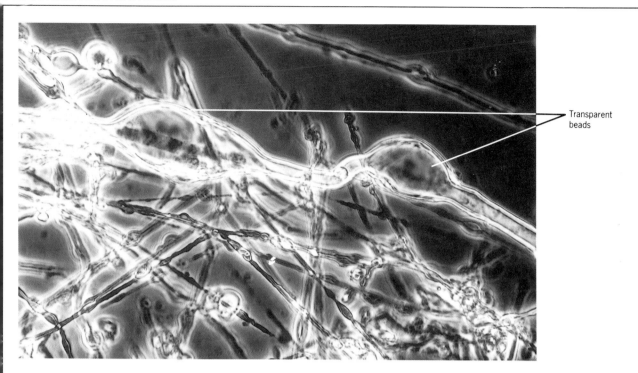

Transparent beads

Figure 128 As previous figure, but showing large beaded fibre (phase contrast, × 700).

The large beads and droplets are transparent.

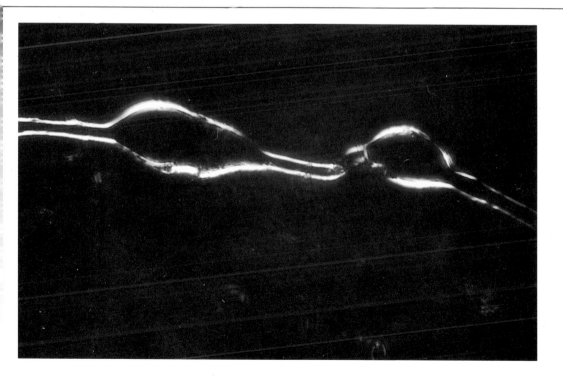

Figure 129 The same fibre as in the previous figure, to show birefringence of the sheath (polarized light, × 700).

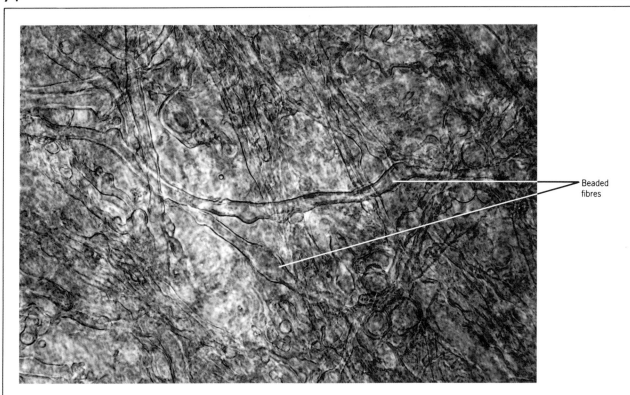

Beaded
fibres

Figure 130   Thin slab of human internal capsule from an 84-year-old male, to show beaded fibres (phase contrast, × 700).

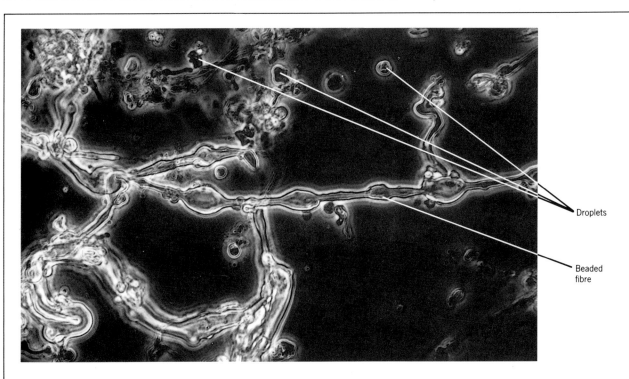

Droplets

Beaded
fibre

Figure 131   As previous figure, but teased to show large beaded fibres and droplets (phase contrast, × 700).
There are granules within the beads.

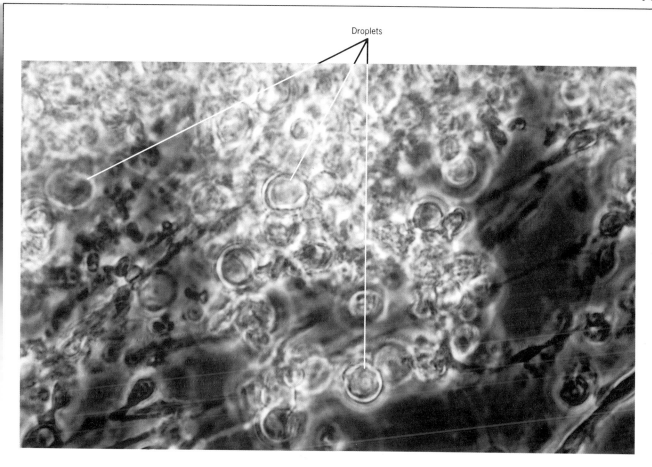

Figure 132   Partially teased rabbit internal capsule, to show large and small droplets (phase contrast, × 2000).

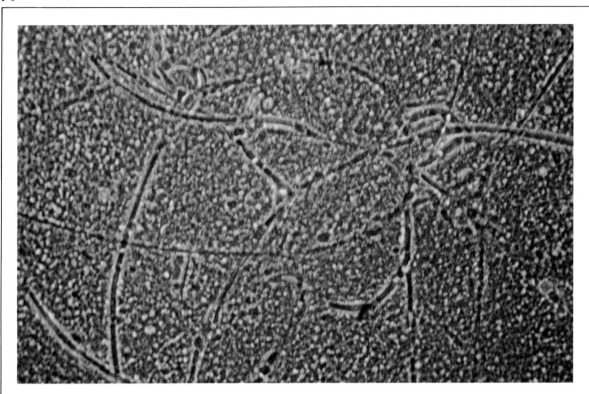

Figure 133   Thin slab of human caudate nucleus from a 65-year-old female, to show blood vessels (phase contrast, × 300).

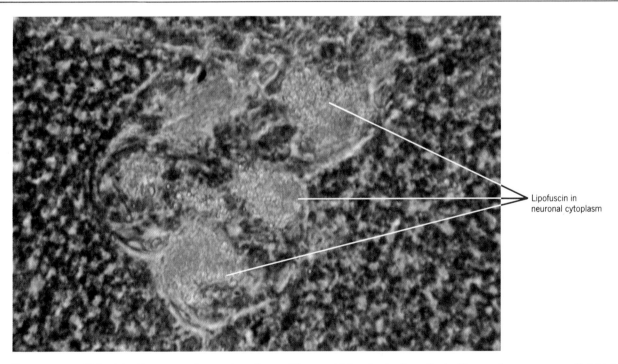

Lipofuscin in
neuronal cytoplasm

Figure 134   Thin slab of human caudate nucleus from a 65-year-old female, to show the incidence of neuron somas (bright field, × 700).

The contrast is given by the lipofuscin.

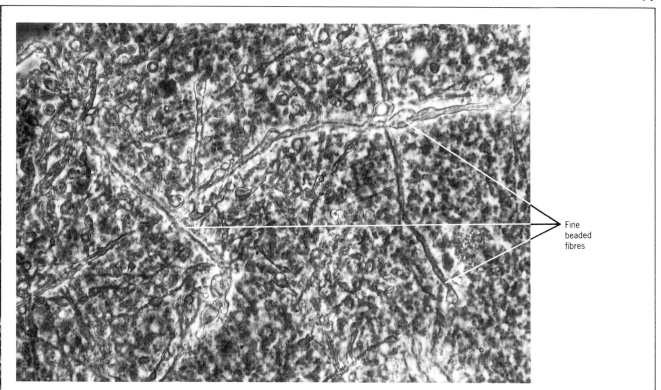

Figure 135 Thin slab of human caudate nucleus from an 80-year-old female, to show fine beaded fibres (phase contrast, × 700).

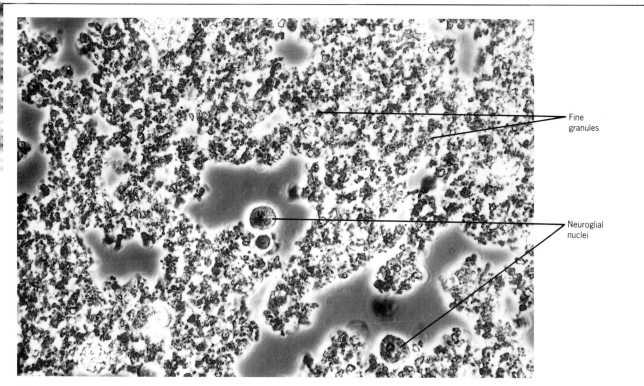

Figure 136 Partially teased human caudate nucleus from a 70-year-old male, to show neuroglial nuclei and fine granules (phase contrast, × 700).

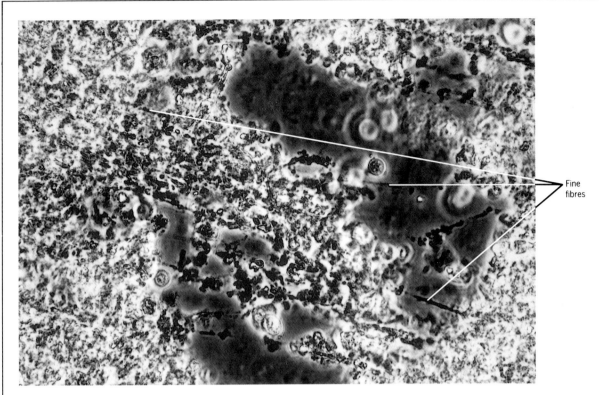

Fine
fibres

Figure 137   As previous specimen, but teased to show fine fibres (phase contrast, × 700).

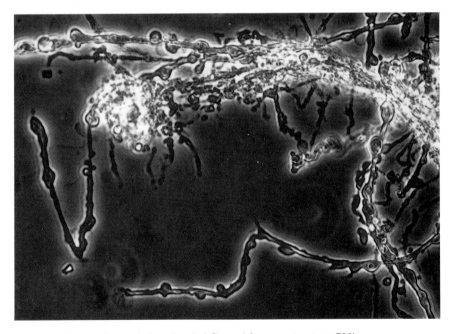

Figure 138   Teased rat caudate nucleus, to show beaded fibres (phase contrast, × 700).

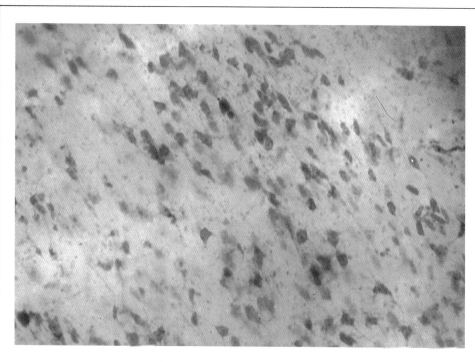

Figure 139 Thin slab of human putamen from a 60-year-old male, lightly coloured with methylene blue to show the incidence of neuron somas (bright field, × 100).

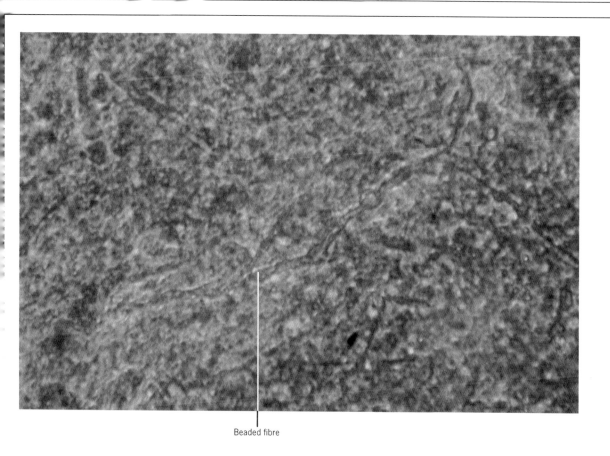

Beaded fibre

Figure 140 Thin slab of human putamen from a 65-year-old female, to show fine beaded fibres (phase contrast, × 720).

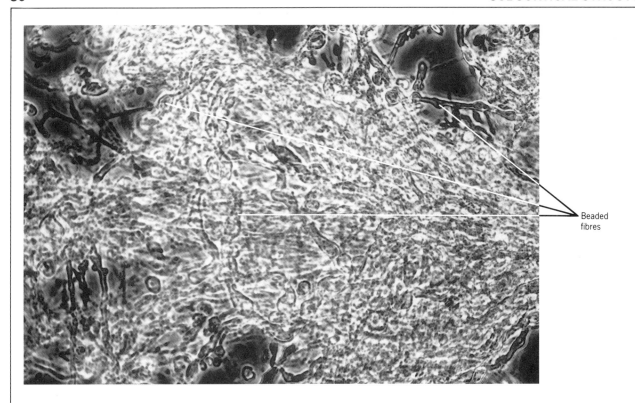

Beaded fibres

Figure 141 Partially teased white matter of a rat putamen, to show beaded fibres (phase contrast, × 700).

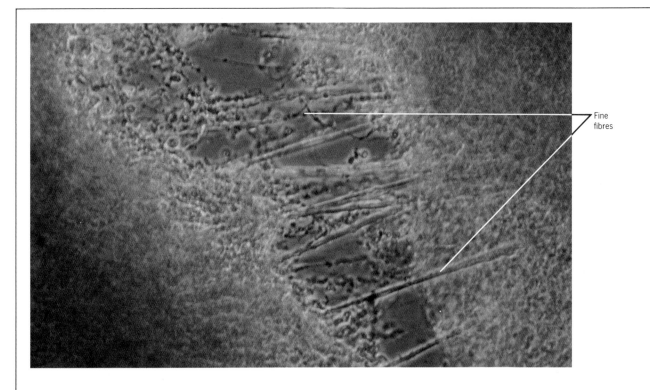

Fine fibres

Figure 142 Teased human putamen from a 65-year-old female, to show fine fibres (phase contrast, × 700).

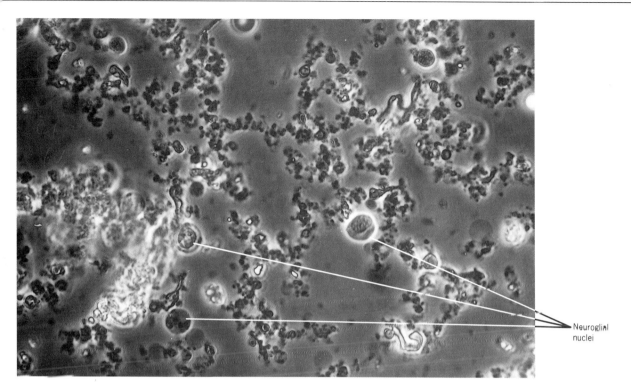

Figure 143   Isolated human neuroglia or small neurons and fine granules from the putamen of a 73-year-old male (phase contrast, × 700).

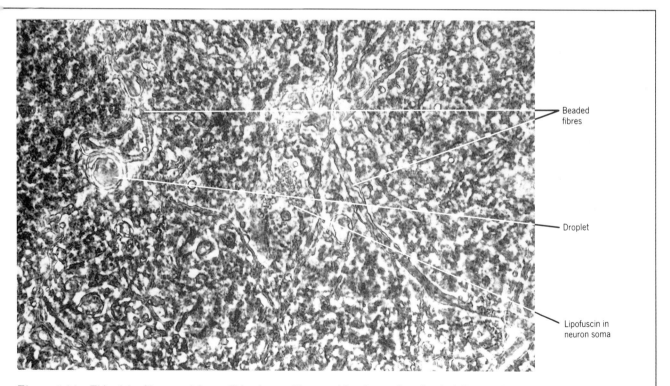

Figure 144   Thin slab of human globus pallidus from a 71-year-old male, to show beaded fibres and a neuron with lipofuscin *in situ* (phase contrast, × 700).

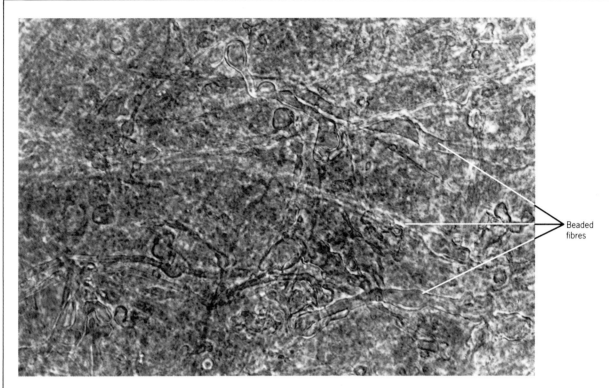

Figure 145   As previous specimen, to show fibres, some beaded (phase contrast, × 700).

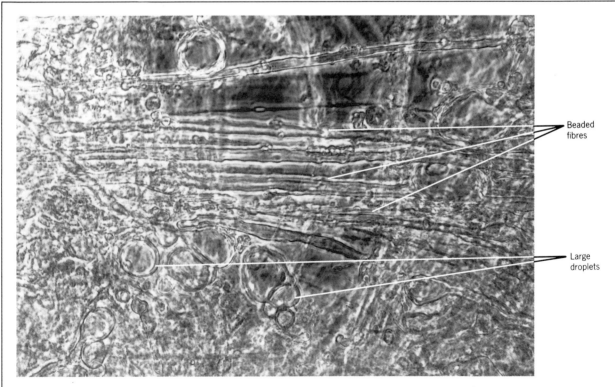

Figure 146   Partially teased human globus pallidus from a 95-year-old female, to show large droplets and fibres (phase contrast, × 700).

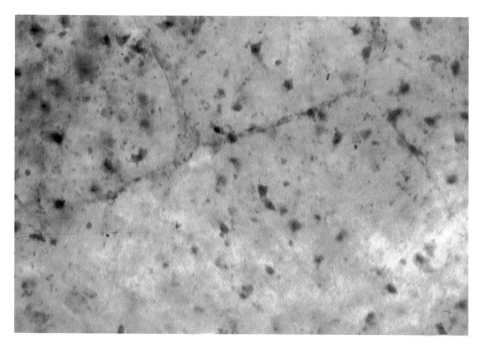

Figure 147 Thin slab of human thalamus from a 60-year-old male, lightly coloured with methylene blue to show the incidence and appearance of neuron somas (bright field, × 100).

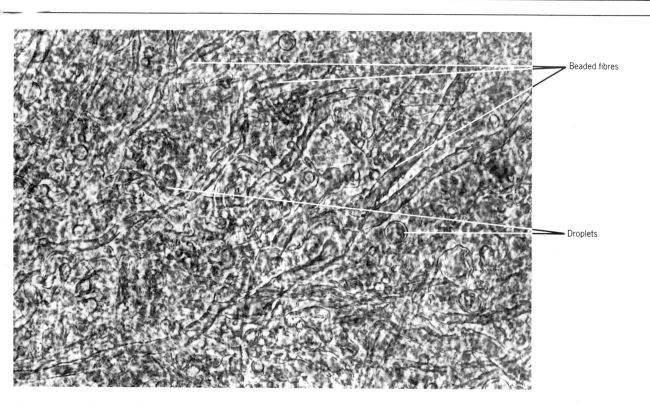

Beaded fibres

Droplets

Figure 148 Thin slab of human dorsolateral nucleus of the thalamus from a 73-year-old male, to show fibres and droplets (phase contrast, × 700).

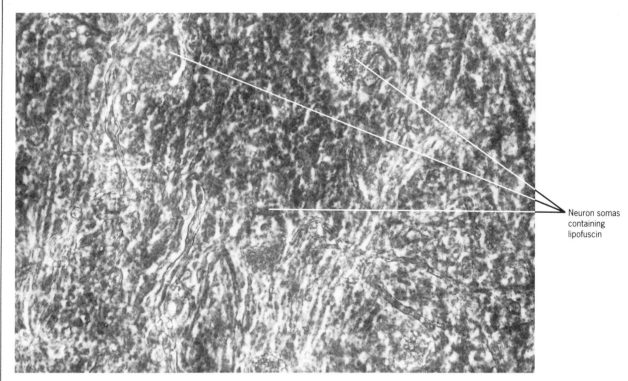

Neuron somas
containing
lipofuscin

Figure 149   Thin slab of human medial nucleus of the thalamus, from a 73-year-old male, to show neurons with intracellular lipofuscin (phase contrast, × 700).

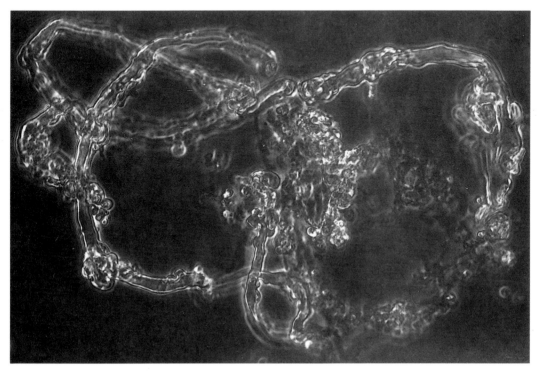

Figure 150   Isolated human beaded fibres from the dorsolateral nucleus of the thalamus from a 73-year-old male (dark ground, × 700).

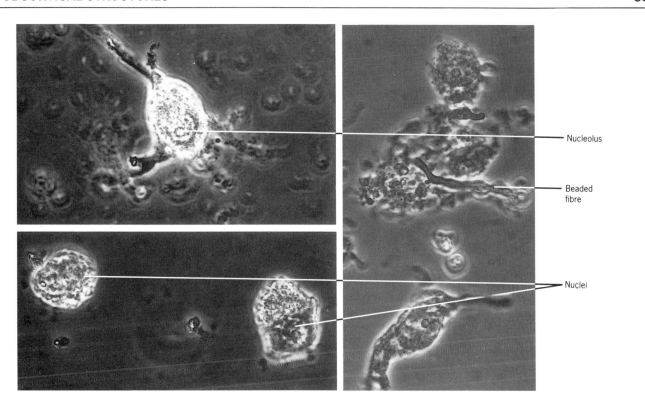

Figure 151   Isolated neurons from thalamus from a 73-year-old human male (left) and from rat (right) (phase contrast, × 700). The dendrites have presumably been detached during teasing of the neurons (bottom left).

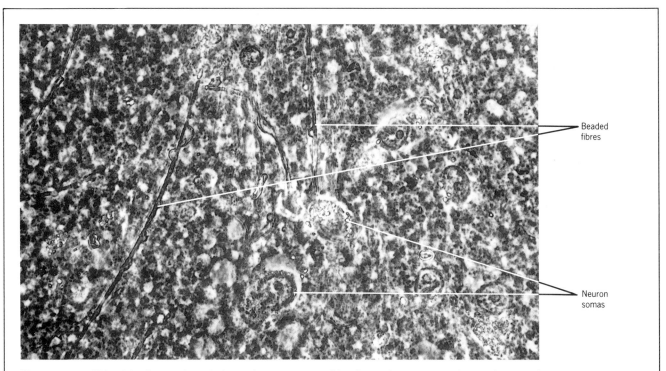

Figure 152   Thin slab of human hypothalamus from a 77-year-old male, to show neuron somas and beaded fibres (phase contrast, × 700).

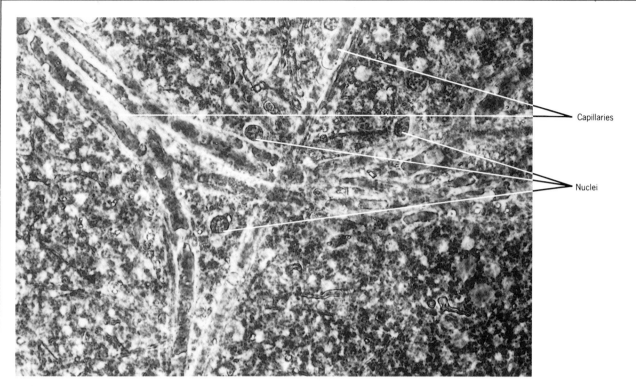

Figure 153   Thin slab of human hypothalamus from a 77-year-old male, to show capillaries and nuclei (phase contrast, × 700).

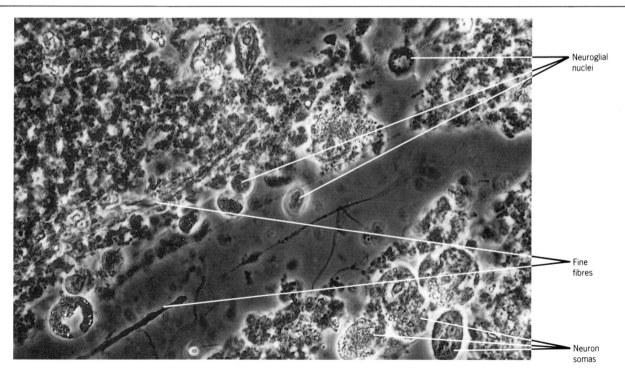

Figure 154   Teased human hypothalamus from a 77-year-old male, to show neurons, fine fibres and neuroglial nuclei (phase contrast, × 700).

The neurons have few or no dendrites.

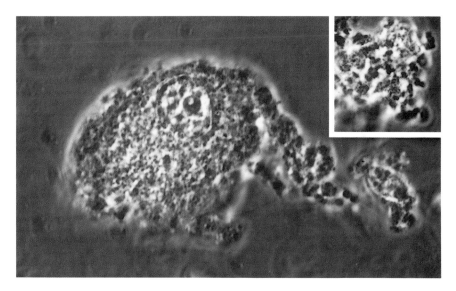

Figure 155 Isolated human hypothalamic neuron from a 53-year-old male (phase contrast, × 1140). Inset: fine granular material adjacent to the latter (phase contrast, × 700).

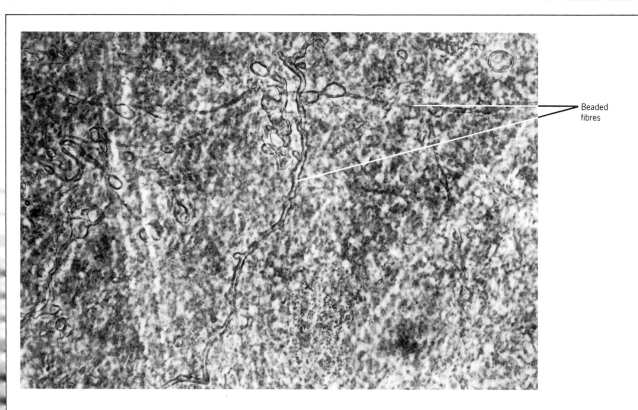

Beaded fibres

Figure 156 Thin slab of human fornix of the hypothalamus from a 77-year-old male, to show beaded fibres (phase contrast, × 700).

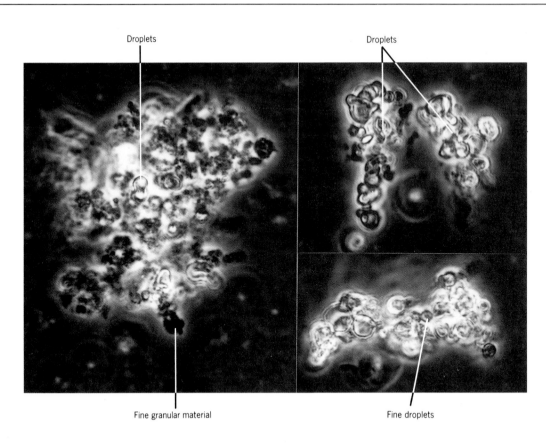

Droplets   Droplets

Fine granular material   Fine droplets

Figure 157   Teased small droplets from previous specimen (phase contrast, × 700).

The droplets are refractile compared with the fine granular material, which is black.

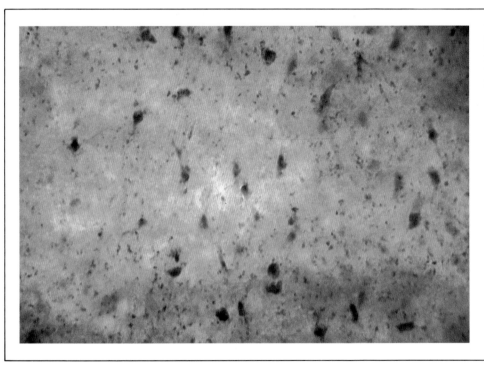

Figure 158   Thin slab of human red nucleus from a 60-year-old male, lightly coloured with methylene blue to show the incidence of neuron somas (bright field, × 100).

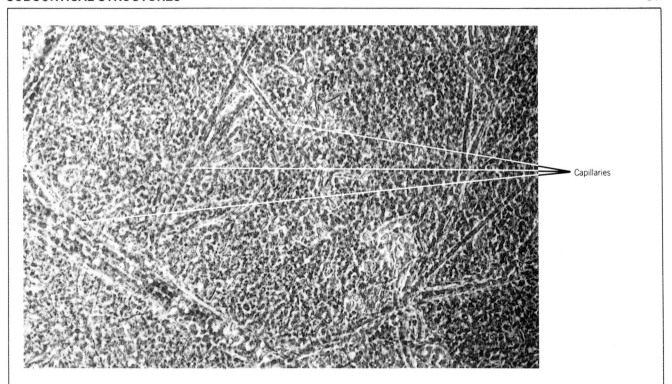

Figure 159   Thin slab of human red nucleus from a 77-year-old male, to show the distribution of capillaries (bright field, × 300).

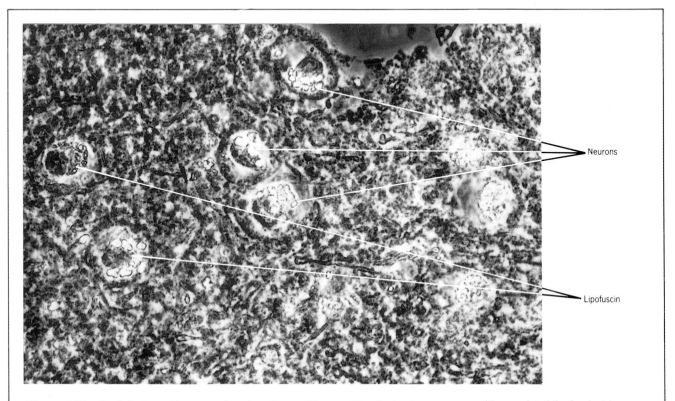

Figure 160   Partially teased human red nucleus from a 77-year-old male, to show neurons with associated lipofuscin (phase contrast, × 700).

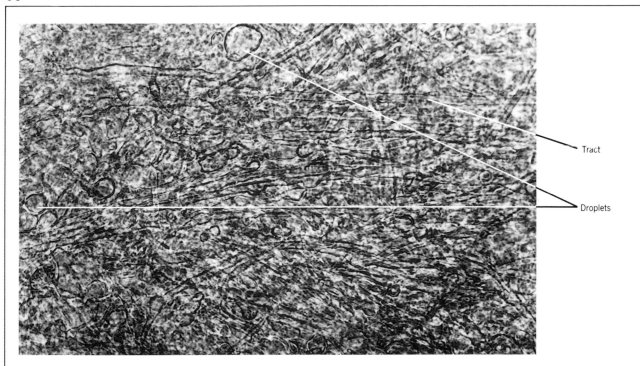

Figure 161   Thin slab of human red nucleus from a 73-year-old male, to show fibre tracts and droplets (phase contrast, × 700).

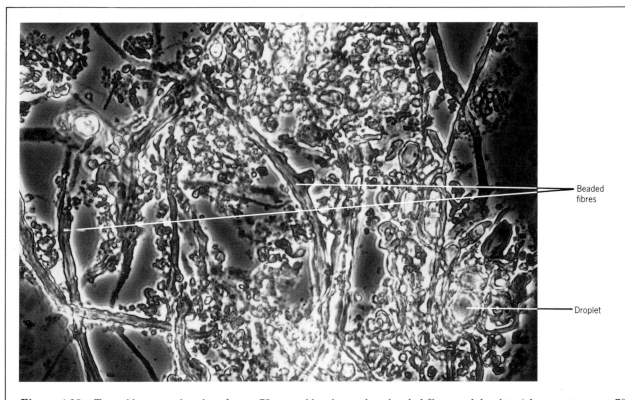

Figure 162   Teased human red nucleus from a 73-year-old male, to show beaded fibres and droplets (phase contrast, × 700).

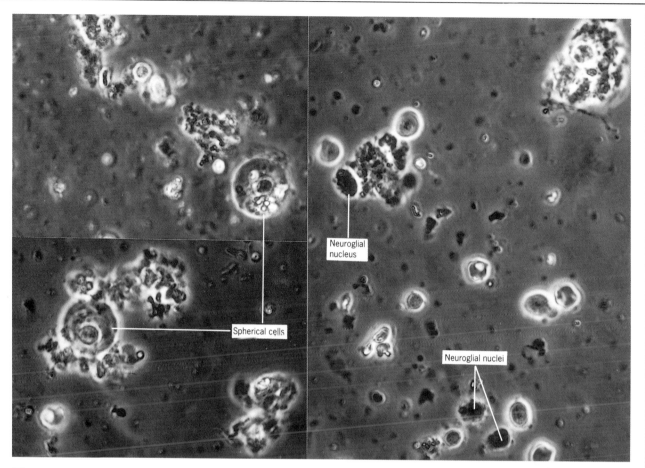

Figure 163 Teased human red nucleus from a 77-year-old male, to show unidentified spherical cells, possible neuron somas and neuroglial nuclei (phase contrast, × 700).

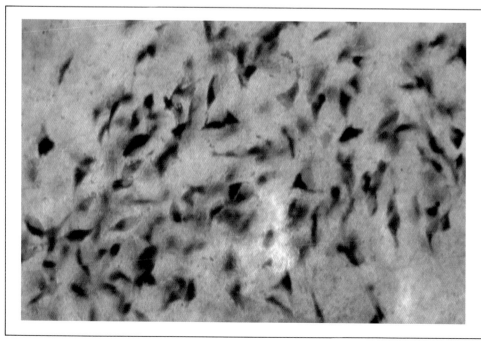

Figure 164 Thin slab of human substantia nigra from a 60-year-old male, lightly coloured with methylene blue to show the high incidence of neuron somas (bright field, × 100).

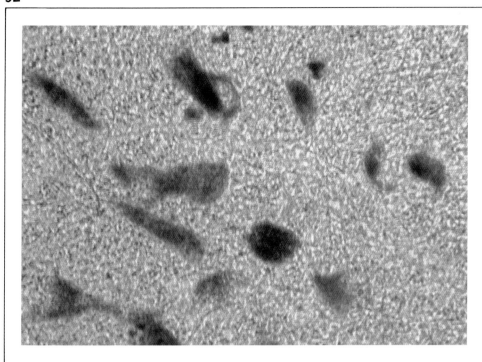

Figure 165 Thin slab of human substantia nigra from an 84-year-old male, to show the incidence of neuron somas (bright field, × 255).

The melanin is naturally brown and in the brain is found only in neurons of the substantia nigra.

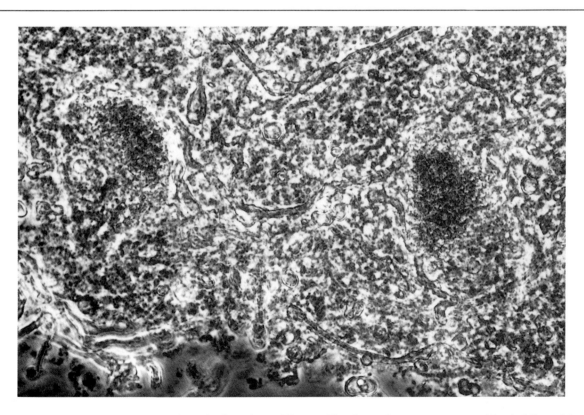

Figure 166 Partially teased human substantia nigra, from a 73-year-old male, to show two neurons and beaded fibres (phase contrast, × 800).

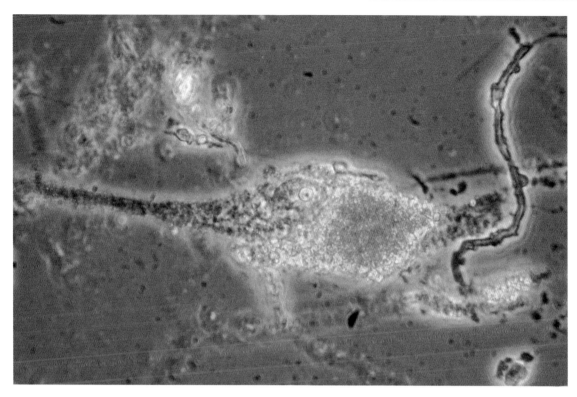

Figure 167 Teased human substantia nigra from a 74-year-old male, to show a neuron with adjacent fine granular material (phase contrast, × 610).

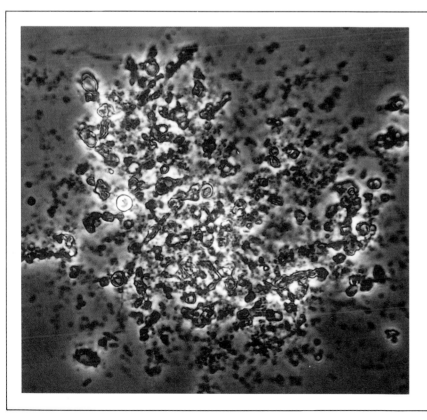

Figure 168 Teased human substantia nigral neuroglia from the previous specimen, to show fine granular material (phase contrast, × 800).

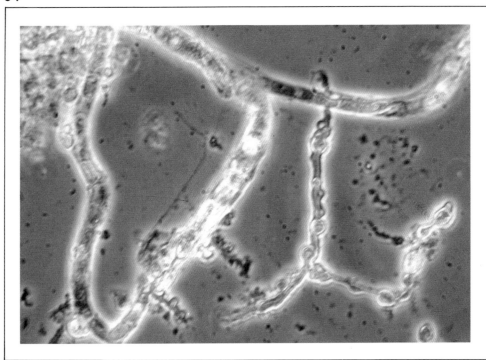

Figure 169 Isolated capillaries and beaded fibres from human substantia nigra of an 84-year-old male (phase contrast, × 610).

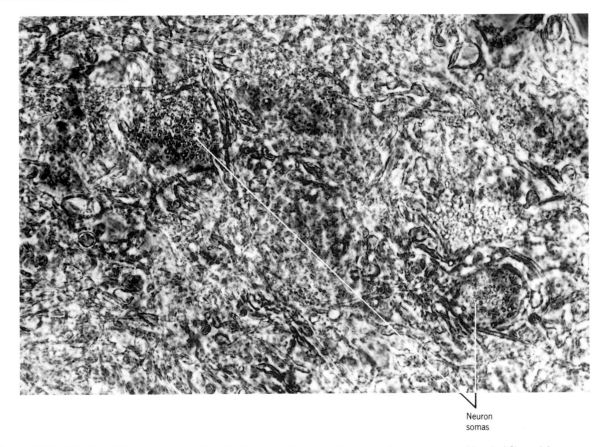

Neuron
somas

Figure 170 Thin slab of the human mammillary body from a 77-year-old male, to show neurons and beaded fibres (phase contrast, × 800).

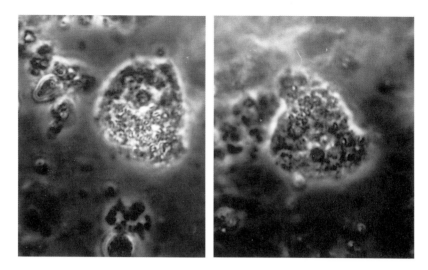

Figure 171   Isolated neuron somas from the previous specimen (phase contrast, × 800).

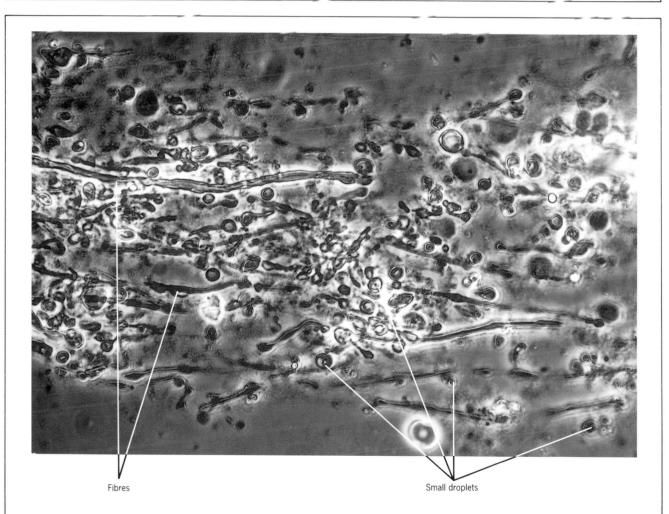

Fibres

Small droplets

Figure 172   Teased fibres and small droplets from the same specimen as in the penultimate figure (phase contrast, × 800).

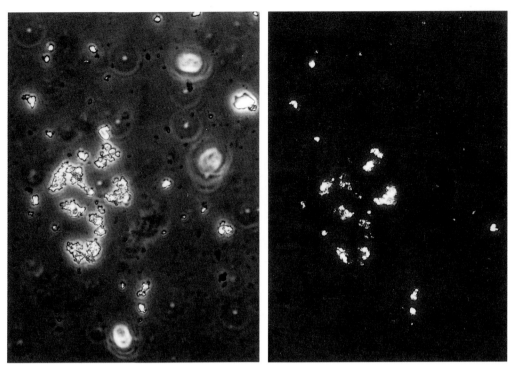

Figure 173   Lipofuscin from the same specimen as in the previous figure, with polars uncrossed (left) and with polars crossed (right) to show birefringence (polarized light, × 700).

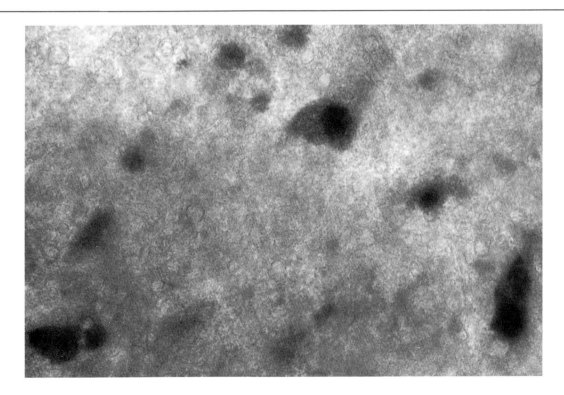

Figure 174   Thin slab of human superior colliculus from a 75-year-old male, lightly coloured with methylene blue to show the incidence of neurons (phase contrast, × 700).

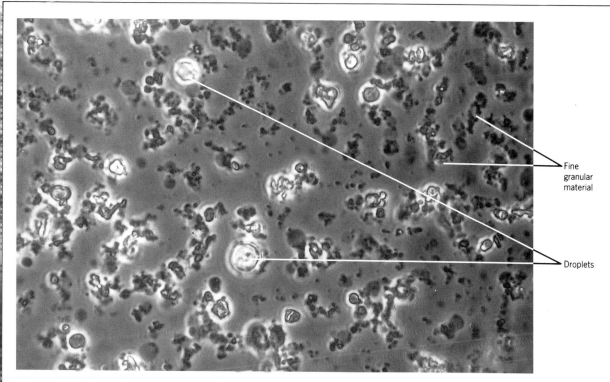

Figure 175 Teased human superior colliculus from a 75-year-old male, to show large refractile droplets and fine granules (phase contrast, × 700).

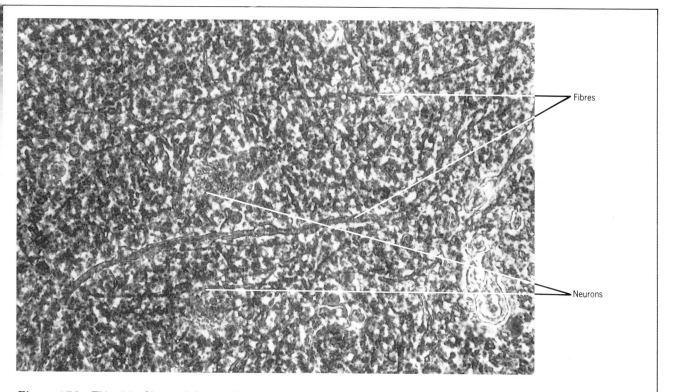

Figure 176 Thin slab of human inferior colliculus from a 75-year-old male (phase contrast, × 700).

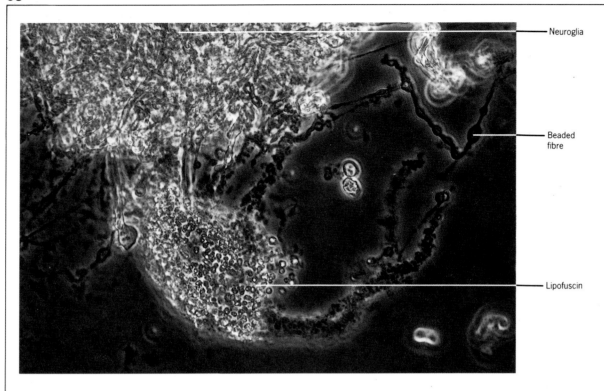

Neuroglia

Beaded fibre

Lipofuscin

Figure 177 Teased human inferior colliculus from a 75-year-old male, to show a neuron covered with lipofuscin and associated neuroglia (phase contrast, × 700).

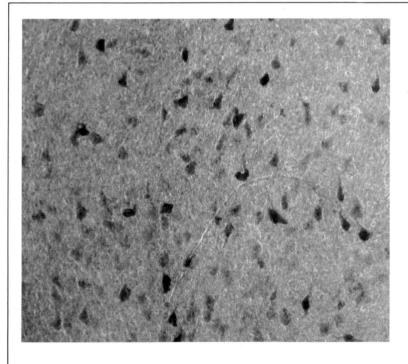

Figure 178 Thin slab of the human hippocampus from a 60-year-old male, lightly coloured with methylene blue to show the incidence of neurons (bright field, × 100).

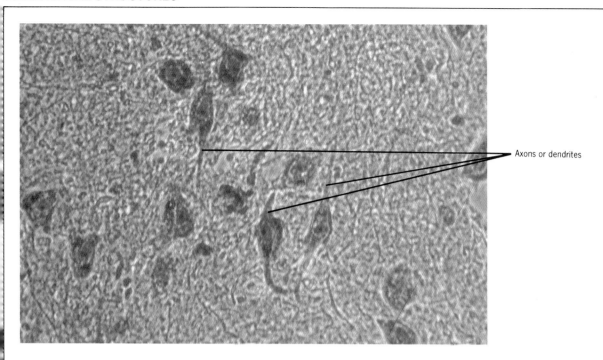

Figure 179 Thin slab of the human hippocampus from a 60-year-old male, lightly coloured with methylene blue to show the incidence and appearance of pyramidal neuron somas (bright field, × 255).

There is lipofuscin in the cytoplasm of some neurons.

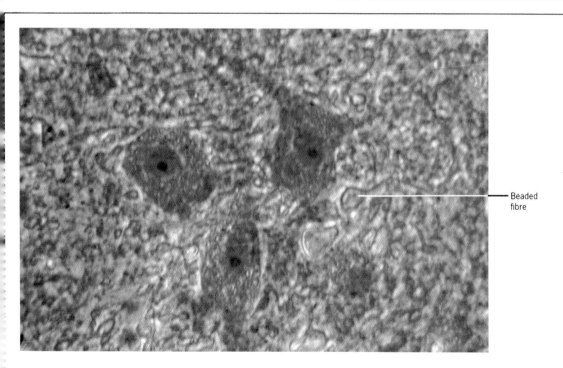

Figure 180 Higher power view of the same specimen as in the previous figure, to show pyramidal neurons *in situ* and fine beaded fibres (bright field, × 610).

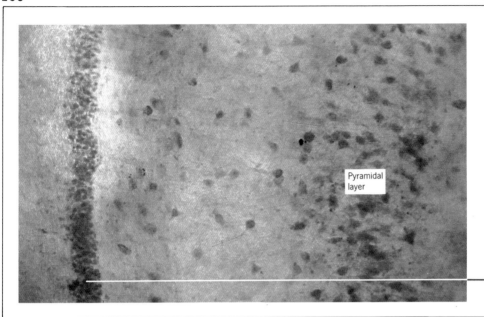

Figure 181 Thin slab of rabbit hippocampus, lightly coloured with methylene blue, to show pyramidal layer (right) and granule cell layer (left) (bright field, × 100).

Pyramidal layer

Granule cell layer

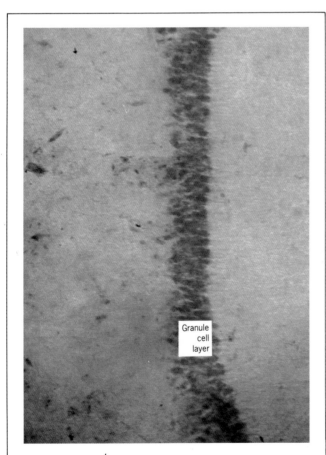

Figure 182 Higher power view of the same specimen as in the previous figure, but enlarged granule cell layer with fine processes proceeding from the cells (bright field, × 255).

Granule cell layer

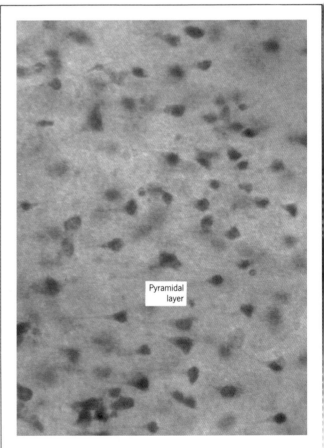

Figure 183 Higher power view of the same specimen as in the previous figure, with the pyramidal cell layer enlarged (bright field, × 255).

The somas of granule cells are smaller than those of the pyramidal neurons.

Pyramidal layer

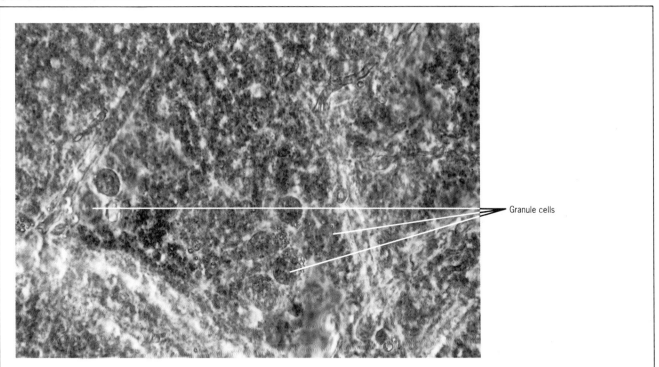

Figure 184   Thin slab of the human hippocampus from an 80-year-old female, to show granule cell somas (phase contrast, × 700).

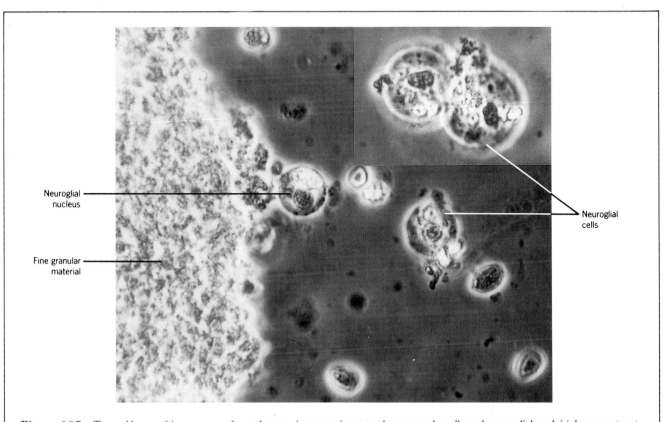

Figure 185   Teased human hippocampus from the previous specimen to show granule cells and neuroglial nuclei (phase contrast, × 700).   Inset : two isolated granule cells.

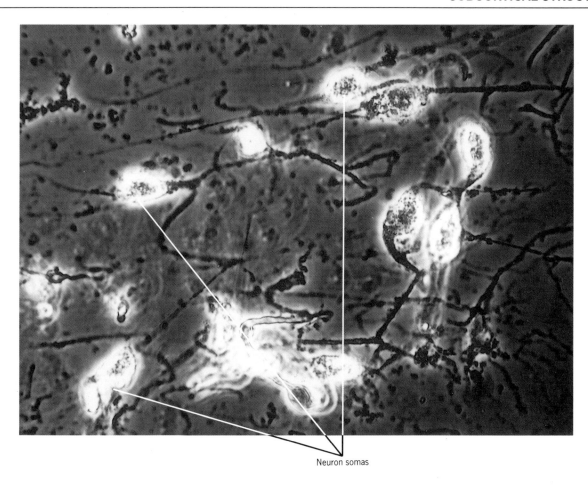

Neuron somas

Figure 186   Teased human hippocampus from a 54-year-old male, to show pyramidal neurons and their processes (phase contrast, × 800).

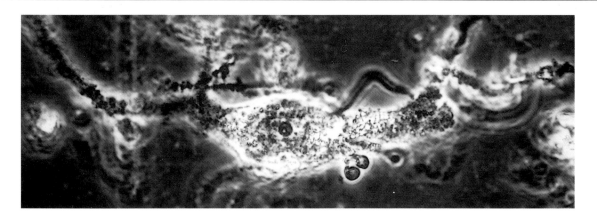

Figure 187   Teased human hippocampal pyramidal neuron from the previous specimen (phase contrast, × 800).

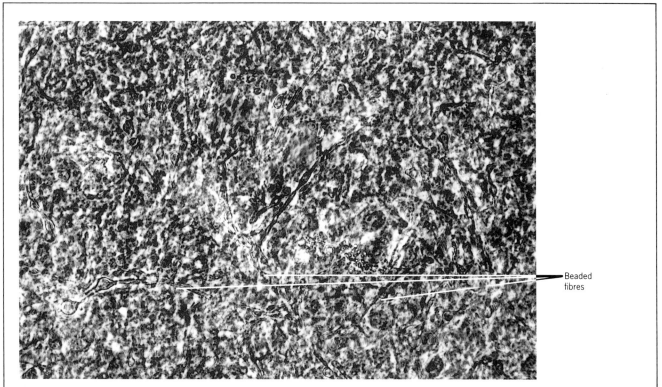

Beaded
fibres

Figure 188   Thin slab of the human amygdala from a 73-year-old male, to show neuron somas and beaded fibres (phase contrast, × 700).

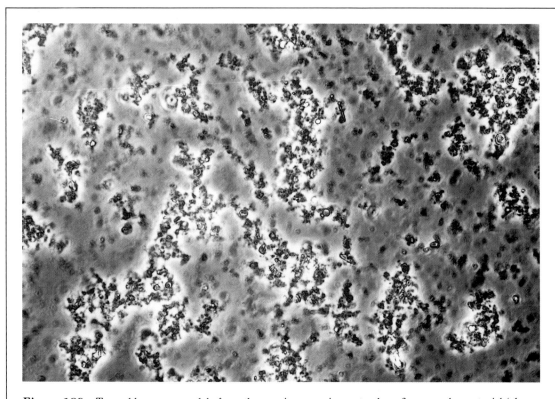

Figure 189   Teased human amygdala from the previous specimen, to show fine granular material (phase contrast, × 700).

Figure 190   Teased human amygdala from the previous specimen, to show round and oval cells and fine granular material (phase contrast, × 800).

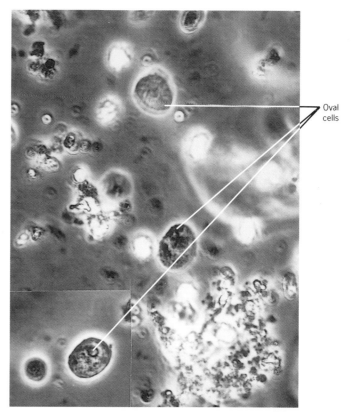

Oval cells

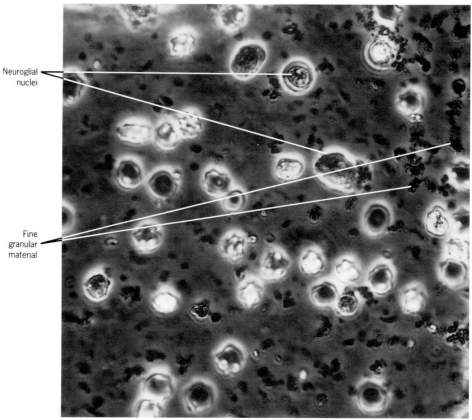

Neuroglial nuclei

Fine granular material

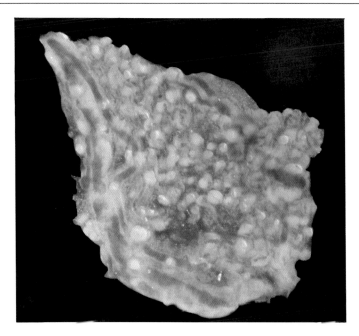

Figure 191 Human choroid plexus from the posterior horn of the lateral ventricle, right side, from a 60-year-old male (bright field, × 15).

The large blood vessels can be seen.

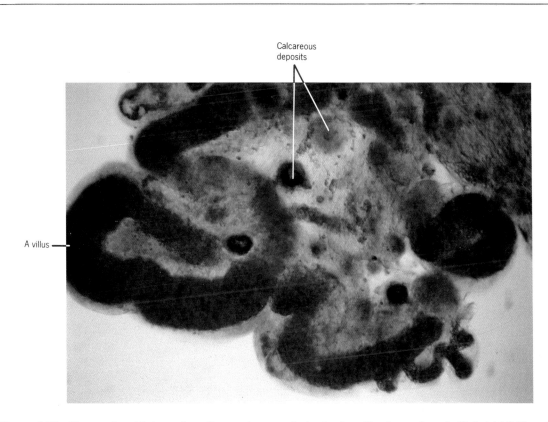

Figure 192 Human choroid plexus from the previous specimen, to show blood vessels and villi (bright field, × 100).

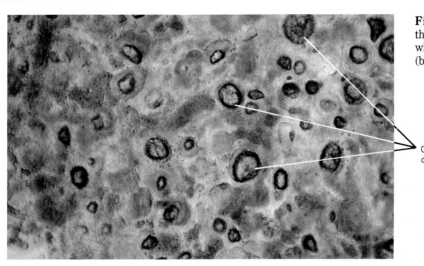

Figure 193   Human choroid plexus from the previous specimen, to show capillaries and what are believed to be calcareous deposits (bright field, × 85).

Calcareous deposits

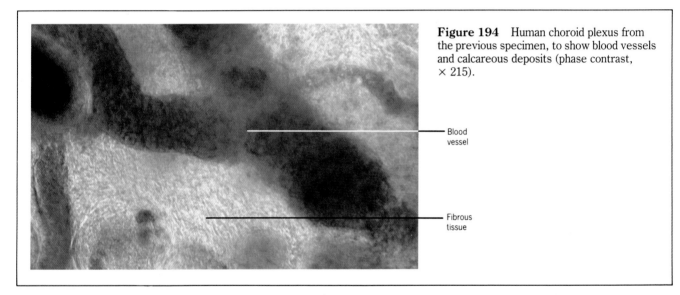

Figure 194   Human choroid plexus from the previous specimen, to show blood vessels and calcareous deposits (phase contrast, × 215).

Blood vessel

Fibrous tissue

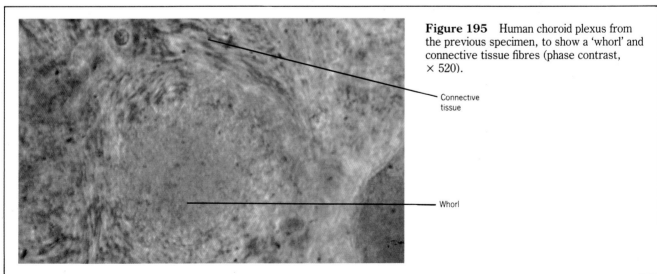

Figure 195   Human choroid plexus from the previous specimen, to show a 'whorl' and connective tissue fibres (phase contrast, × 520).

Connective tissue

Whorl

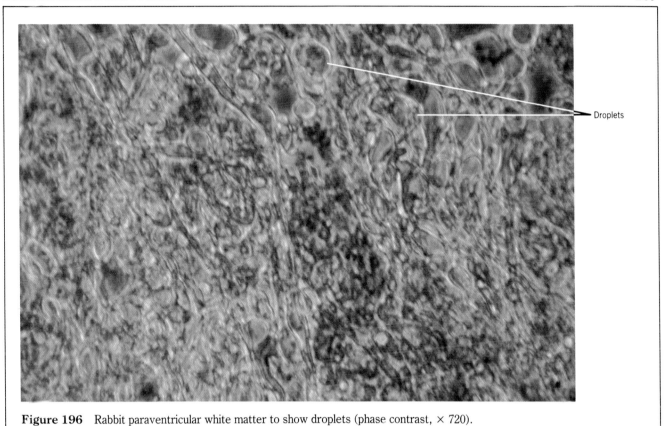

Figure 196   Rabbit paraventricular white matter to show droplets (phase contrast, × 720).

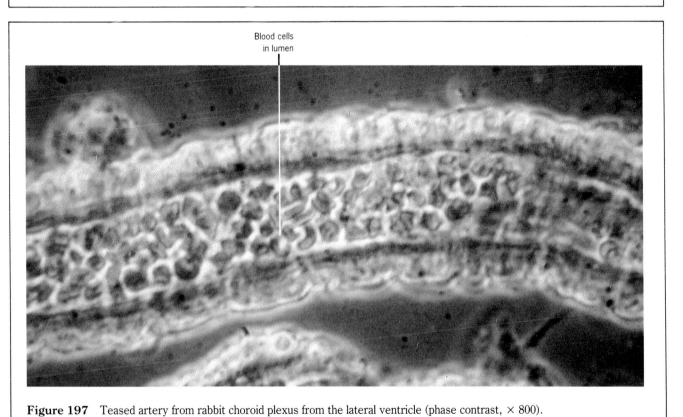

Figure 197   Teased artery from rabbit choroid plexus from the lateral ventricle (phase contrast, × 800).

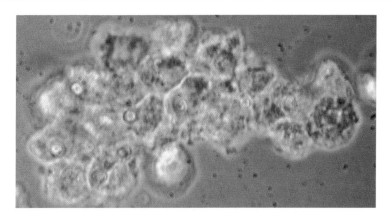

Figure 198 Isolated human epithelial cells from the choroid plexus of a 60-year-old male (phase contrast, × 600).

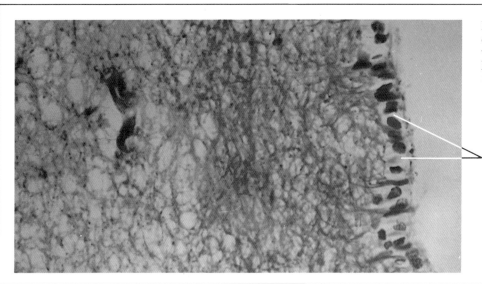

Figure 199 Human ependymal cells and adjacent white matter stained with Holzer's stain (bright field, × 600).

Ependymal cells

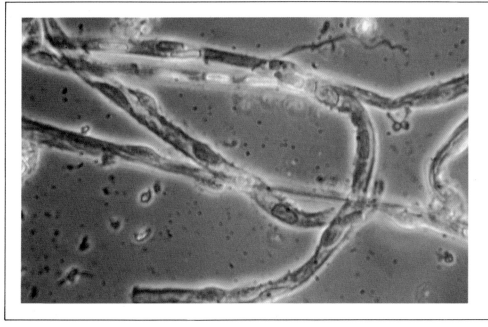

Figure 200 Rabbit capillary from the white matter adjacent to the third ventricle (phase contrast, × 600).

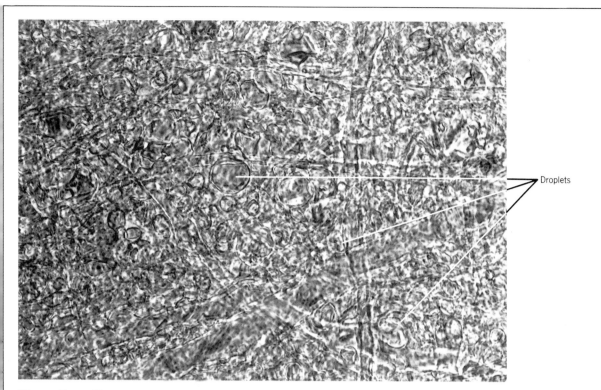

Figure 201 Thin slab of human pyramid from a 95-year-old female, to show fibres and large and small droplets (phase contrast, × 700).

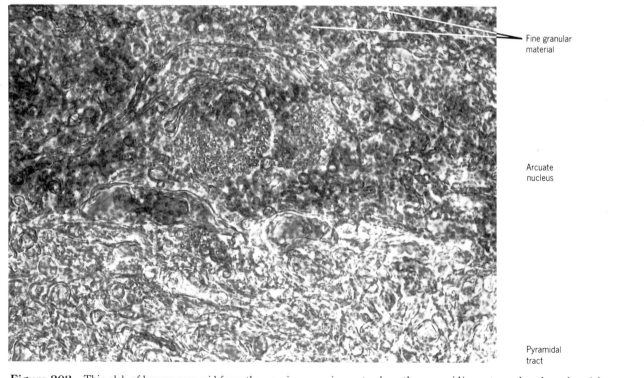

Figure 202 Thin slab of human pyramid from the previous specimen, to show the pyramid/arcuate nucleus boundary (phase contrast, × 700).

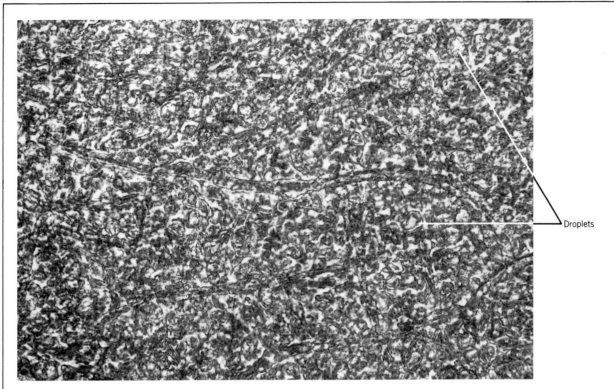

Figure 203   Thin slab of human pons from a 95-year-old female, to show beaded fibres and droplets (phase contrast, × 700).

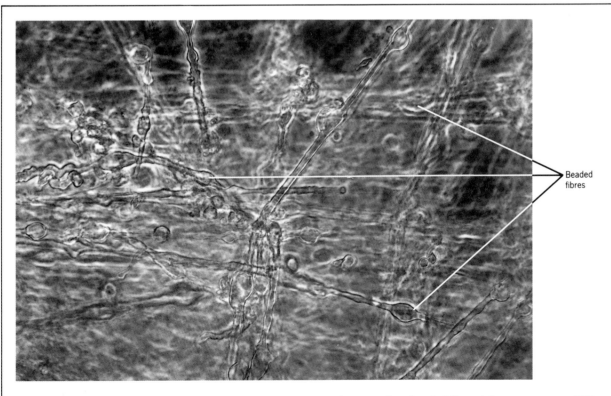

Figure 204   Partially teased human pons from the previous specimen, to show beaded fibres (phase contrast, × 700).

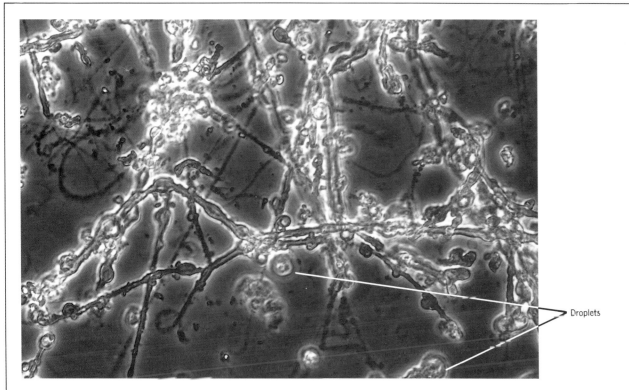

Droplets

Figure 205 Teased human pons from the previous specimen, to show beaded fibres and droplets (phase contrast, × 700).

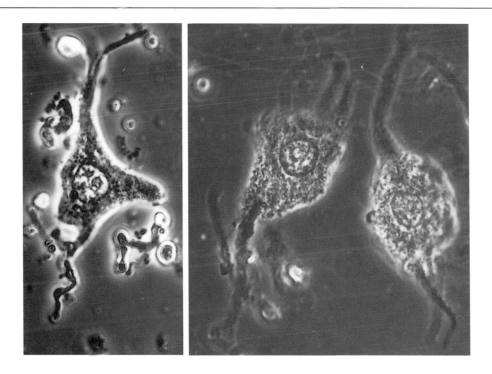

Figure 206 Isolated neurons from the teased human pontine nucleus from a 54-year-old male (phase contrast, × 700).

Note how small these neurons are.

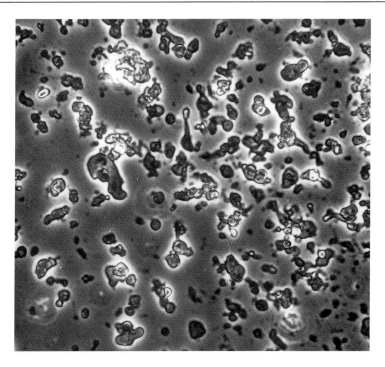

Figure 207 Teased guinea-pig pons to show refractile droplets (phase contrast, × 700).

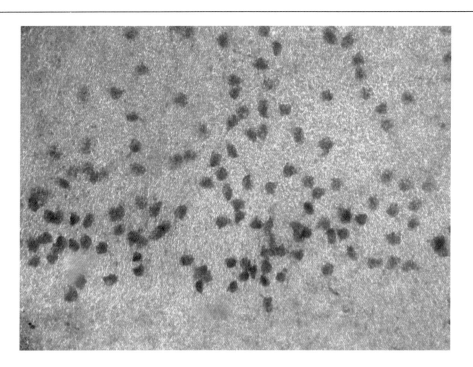

Figure 208 Thin slab of human olivary nucleus from a 60-year-old male, lightly coloured with methylene blue to show the incidence of neuron somas (bright field, × 100).

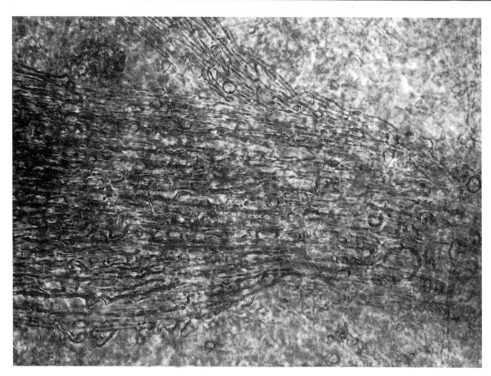

Figure 209   Thin slab of human olivary nucleus from a 77-year-old male, to show a fibre tract *in situ* (phase contrast, × 700).

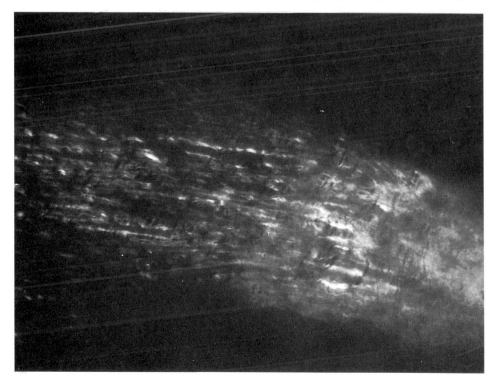

Figure 210   The same thin slab of human olivary nucleus as in the previous specimen, to show birefringence of some fibres (polarized light, × 700).

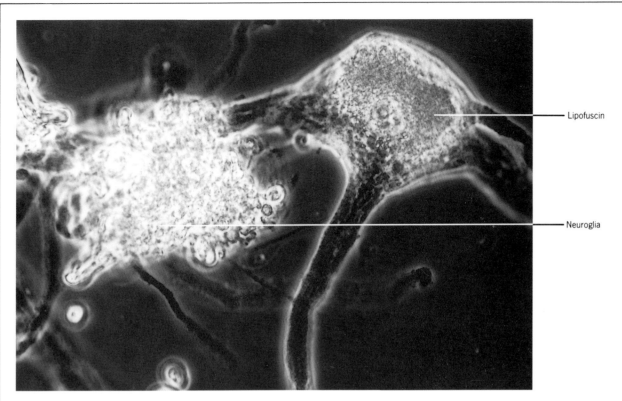

Lipofuscin

Neuroglia

Figure 211   Isolated neuron from teased human olivary nucleus from a 77-year-old male, with adherent neuroglia (phase contrast, × 700).

The neuron soma is more than half full of lipofuscin.

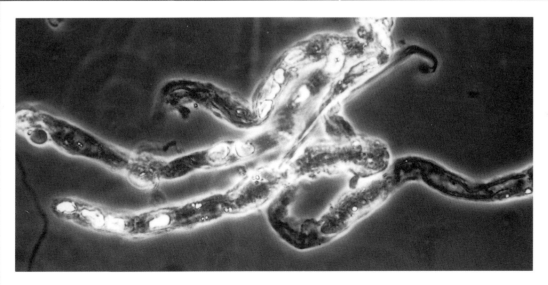

Figure 212   Isolated capillaries from teased human olivary nucleus from a 77-year-old male (phase contrast, × 700).

Note the thinness of the walls.

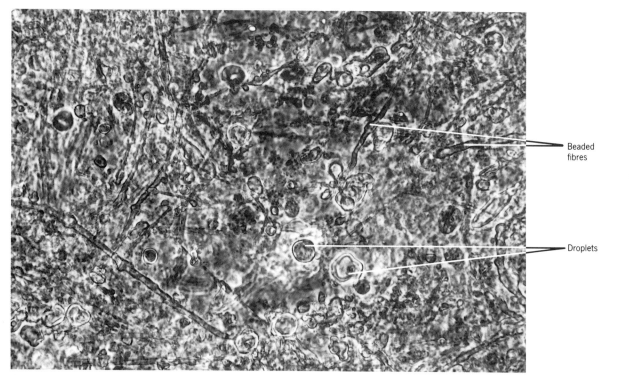

Figure 213 Thin slab of human medial lemniscus from a 95-year-old female, to show beaded fibres and droplets (phase contrast, × 700).

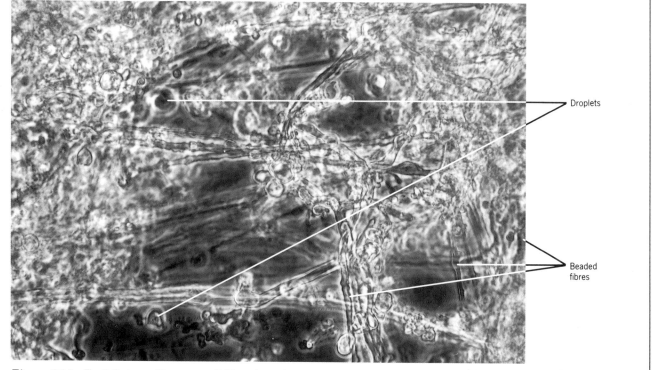

Figure 214 Partially teased human medial lemniscus from the previous specimen, to show beaded fibres and droplets (phase contrast, × 700).

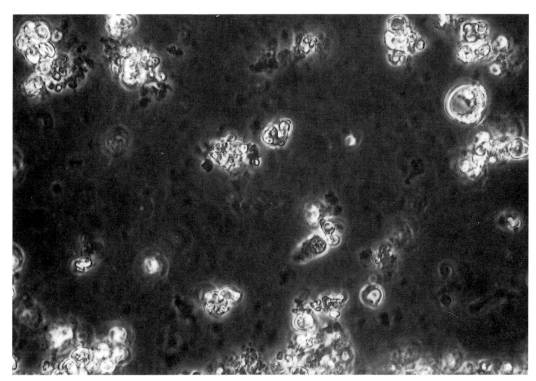

Figure 215   Teased human medial lemniscus from the previous specimen, to show isolated droplets (phase contrast, × 700).

These droplets appear refractile and transparent compared with granules, which are dark.

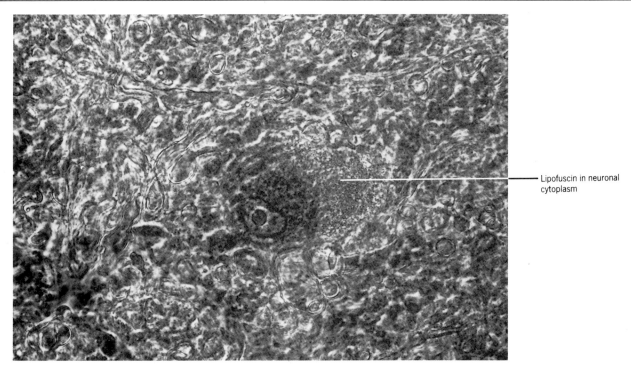

Lipofuscin in neuronal cytoplasm

Figure 216   Thin slab of human inferior vestibular nucleus from a 68-year-old male, to show a neuron with lipofuscin *in situ* and beaded fibres (phase contrast, × 700).

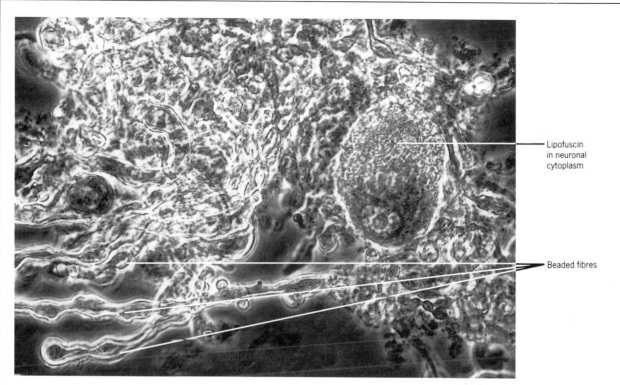

Figure 217 Partially teased human inferior vestibular nucleus from the previous specimen to show neuron and beaded fibres (phase contrast, × 700).

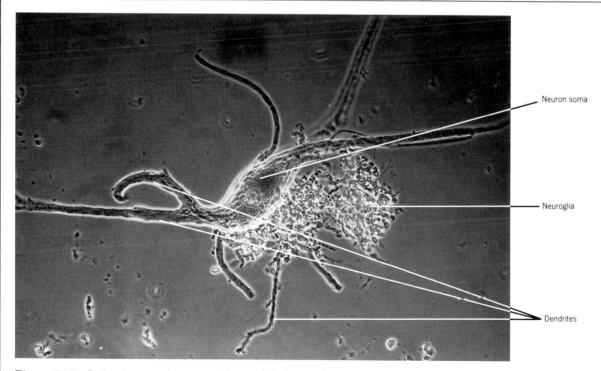

Figure 218 Isolated neuron from teased human inferior vestibular nucleus from a 53-year-old male, with adherent neuroglia (phase contrast, × 280).

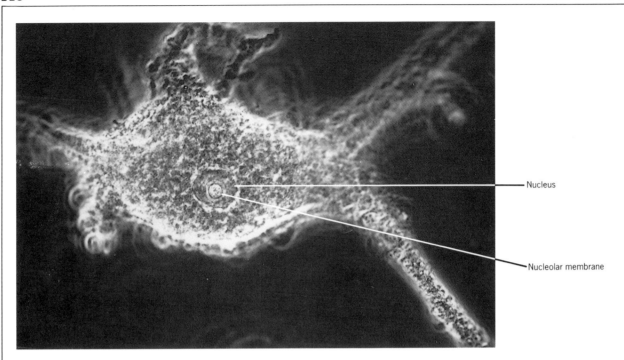

Figure 219   Isolated rabbit neuron from teased lateral vestibular nucleus to show nuclear and nucleolar membranes (phase contrast, × 700).

The nucleolar membrane is seen when the somas are dissected out in saline, but not in sucrose (Hussain *et al.*, 1974).

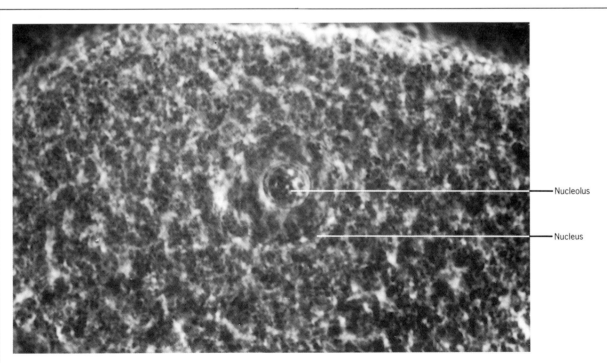

Figure 220   Isolated rabbit neuron soma from teased lateral vestibular nucleus, to show details of nucleolus (phase contrast, × 2000).

The nucleolonema moves during life (Sartory *et al.*, 1971).

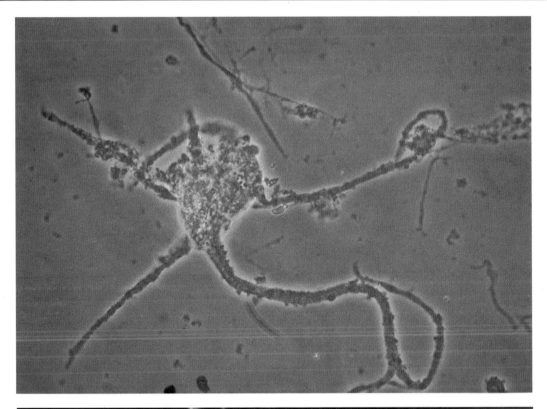

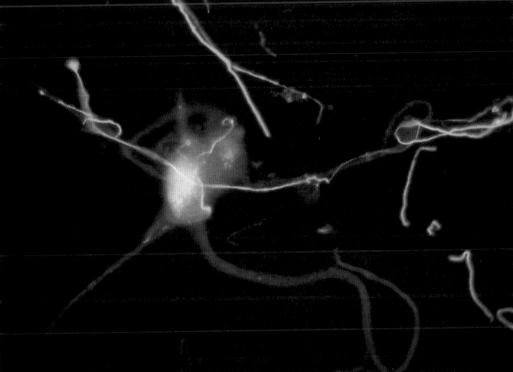

Figure 221   Isolated human neuron from the lateral vestibular nucleus of an 82-year-old male, stained with anti-neurofilament 200 kD protein, by phase contrast (above) and after excitation with blue light of 450–490 nm (below) ($\times$ 500).

Fibres probably unmyelinated can be seen fluorescing, but the fine granular material does not.

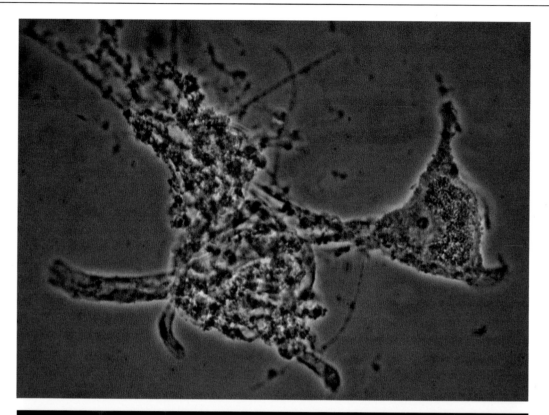

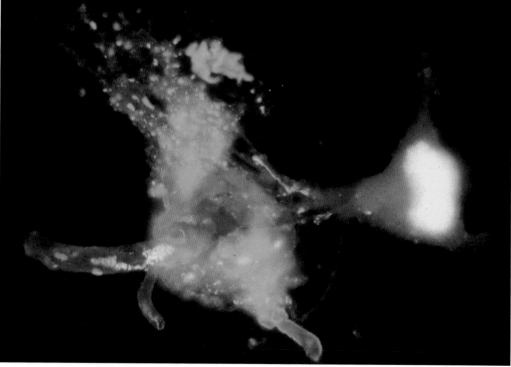

Figure 222 Isolated human neuron from the lateral vestibular nucleus of a 64-year-old male, stained with anti-glial fibrillary acidic protein, by phase contrast (above) and after excitation with blue light of 450–490 nm (below) ($\times$ 500).

Some fine granules can be seen fluorescing, compare with the previous figure.

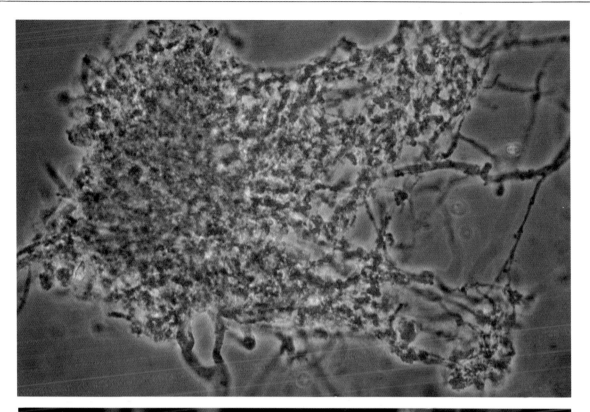

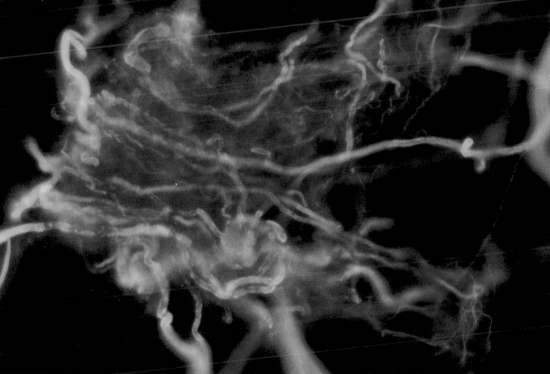

Figure 223 Isolated human neuroglia from the lateral vestibular nucleus of an 82-year-old male, stained with anti-neurofilament 200 kD protein, by phase contrast (above) and after excitation with blue light of 450–490 nm (below) (× 500).

The lipofuscin fluoresces brightly, as do probably unmyelinated fibres, but the main dendrites only weakly.

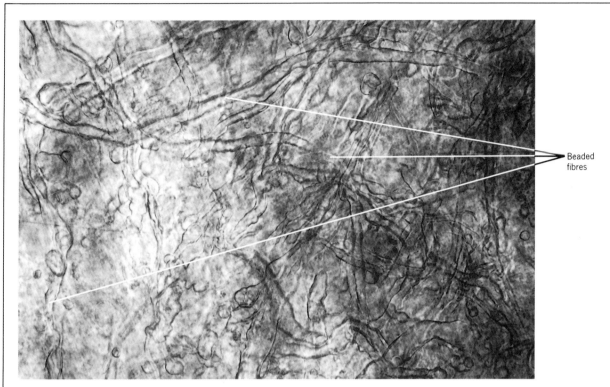

Figure 224   Thin slab of human medullary white matter from a 95-year-old female, to show beaded fibres *in situ* (phase contrast, × 700).

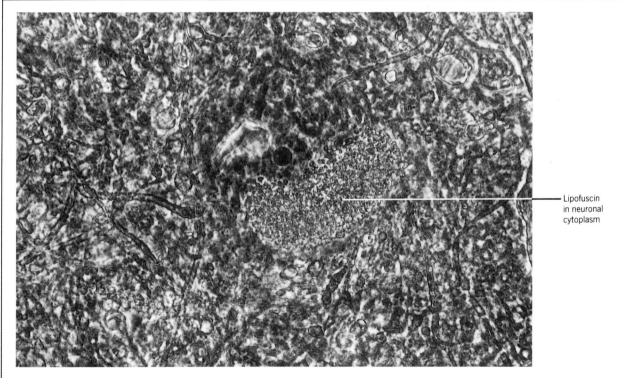

Figure 225   Thin slab of human dorsal nucleus of the vagus from a 95-year-old female, to show a neuron *in situ* with large lipofuscin deposit (phase contrast, × 700).

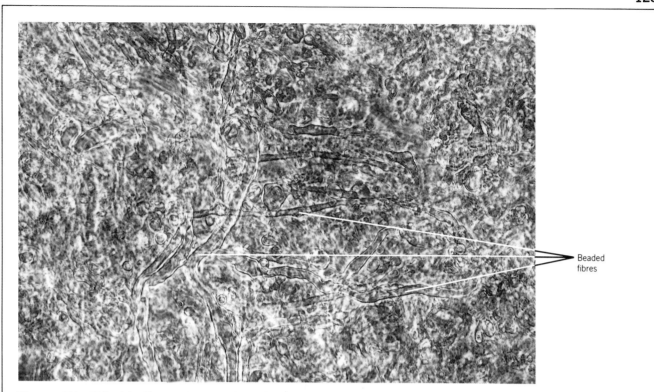

Beaded
fibres

Figure 226 Thin slab of human dorsal nucleus of the vagus from a 95-year-old female, to show beaded fibres *in situ* (phase contrast, × 700).

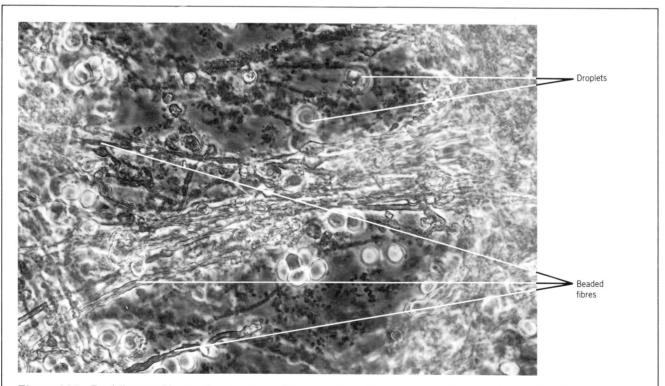

Droplets

Beaded
fibres

Figure 227 Partially teased human dorsal nucleus of the vagus from the previous specimen, to show beaded fibres (phase contrast, × 700).

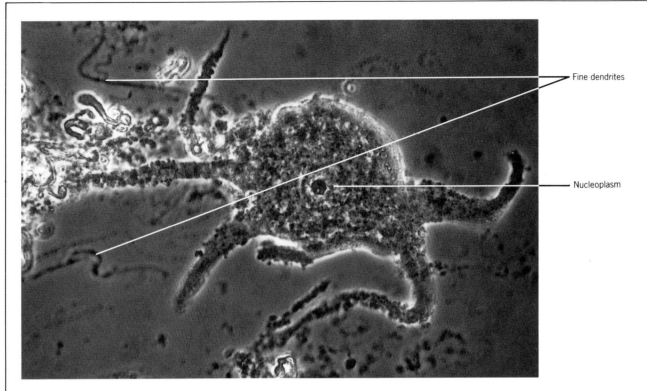

Fine dendrites

Nucleoplasm

Figure 228   Isolated neuron from the dorsal nucleus of the vagus from a 53-year-old male (phase contrast, × 700).

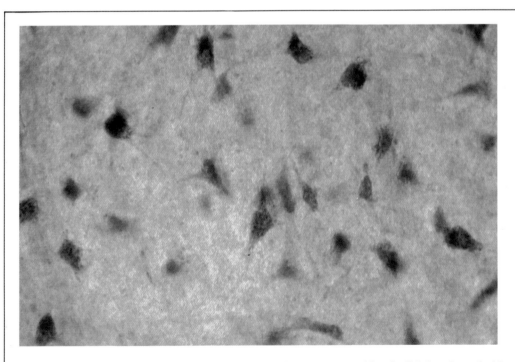

Figure 229   Thin slab of human hypoglossal nucleus from a 60-year-old male, lightly coloured with methylene blue to show the incidence and appearance of neuron somas (bright field, × 100).

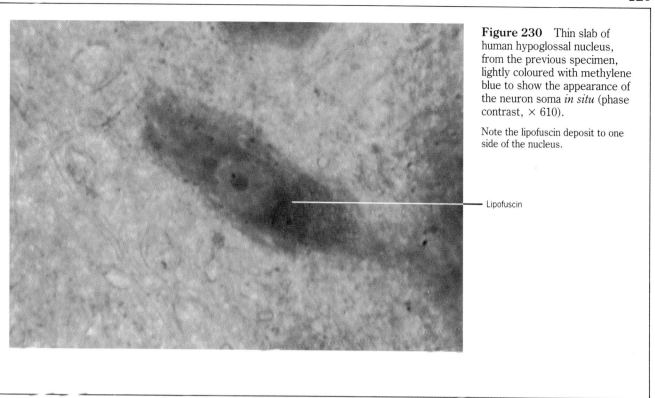

Figure 230 Thin slab of human hypoglossal nucleus, from the previous specimen, lightly coloured with methylene blue to show the appearance of the neuron soma *in situ* (phase contrast, × 610).

Note the lipofuscin deposit to one side of the nucleus.

— Lipofuscin

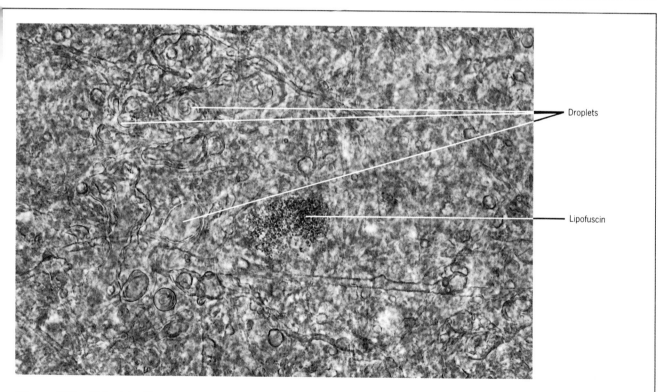

Droplets

Lipofuscin

Figure 231 Thin slab of human hypoglossal nucleus, from a 95-year-old female, to show lipofuscin, beaded fibres and droplets (phase contrast, × 700).

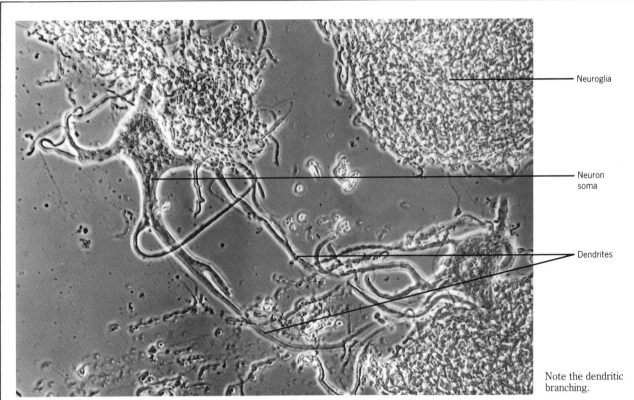

Neuroglia

Neuron
soma

Dendrites

Note the dendritic
branching.

Figure 232   Teased human hypoglossal nucleus from a 62-year-old female, to show neurons and neuroglia (phase contrast, × 300).

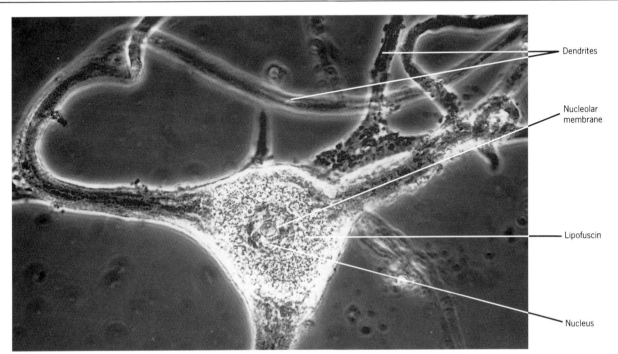

Dendrites

Nucleolar
membrane

Lipofuscin

Nucleus

Figure 233   Isolated human neuron from the hypoglossal nucleus of the previous specimen (phase contrast, × 700).

Near the soma, it is usually difficult to distinguish with certainty between small primary dendrites and axons.

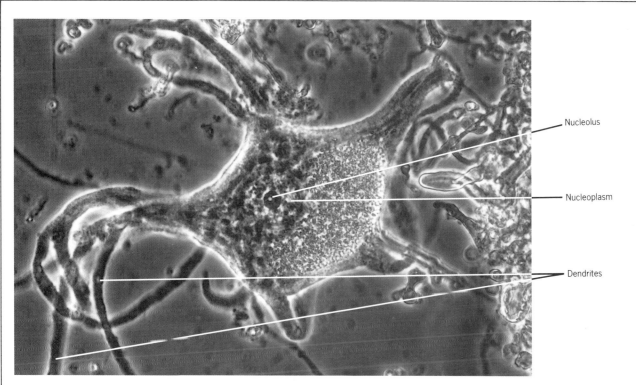

Nucleolus

Nucleoplasm

Dendrites

Figure 234 Isolated human neuron from the hypoglossal nucleus of the previous specimen (phase contrast, × 700).

Note the dense material in the cytoplasm and dendrites.

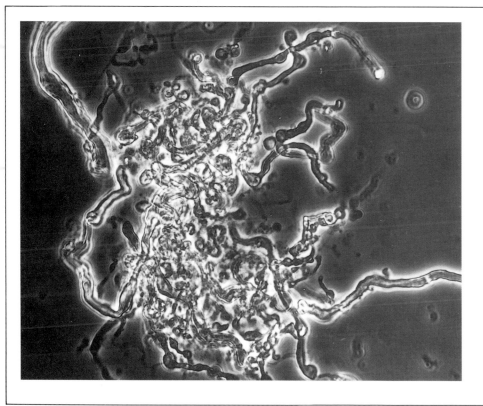

Figure 235 Teased human white matter adjacent to the hypoglossal nucleus of a 62-year-old female, to show beaded fibres (phase contrast, × 700).

SECTION 5

CEREBELLUM

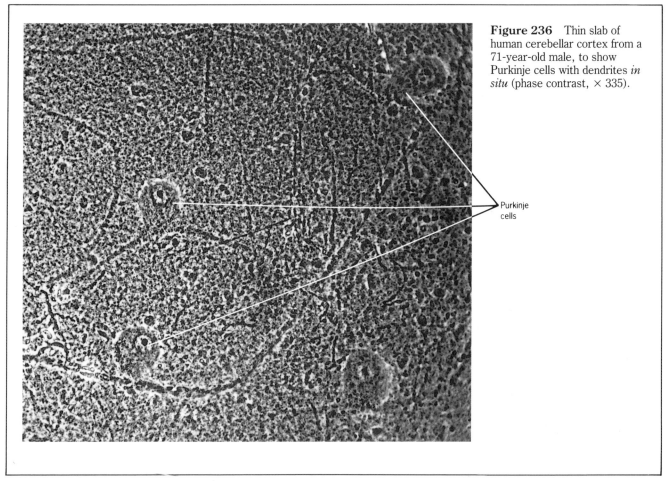

Figure 236 Thin slab of human cerebellar cortex from a 71-year-old male, to show Purkinje cells with dendrites *in situ* (phase contrast, × 335).

Purkinje cells

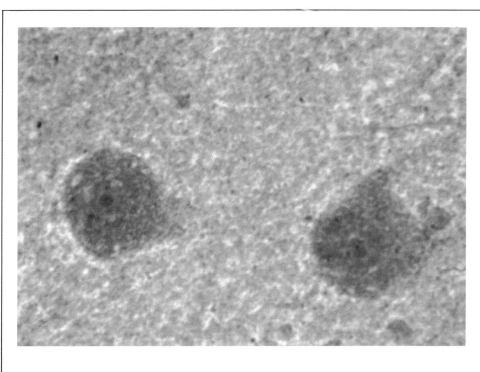

Figure 237 Thin slab of human cerebellar cortex from an 84-year-old male, lightly coloured with methylene blue to show Purkinje cell somas *in situ* (bright field, × 610).

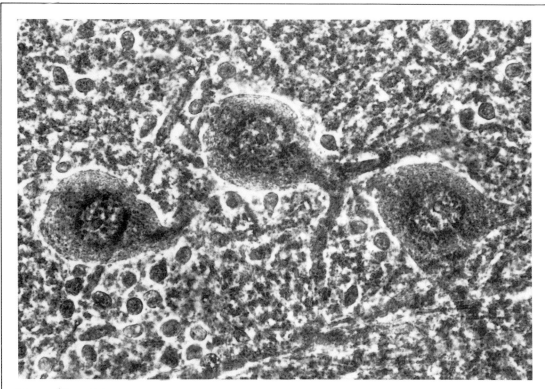

Figure 238 Thin slab of lamb cerebellar cortex to show Purkinje and granule cells *in situ* (phase contrast, × 700).

These cells were originally described by Purkinje in 1838.

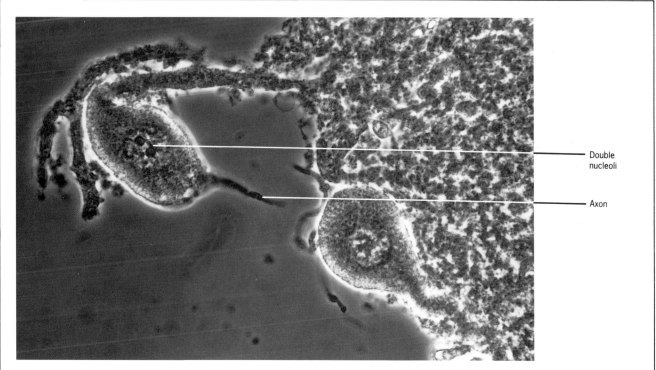

Double nucleoli

Axon

Figure 239 Partially teased lamb cerebellar cortex to show two Purkinje cells, one with two nucleoli and associated neuroglia (phase contrast, × 700).

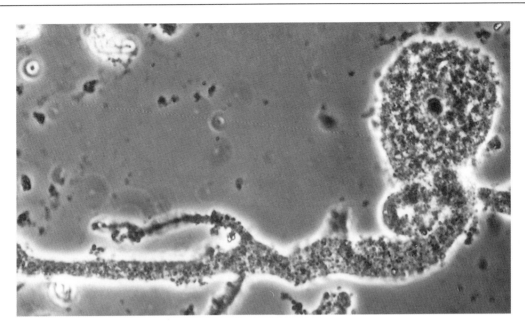

Figure 240   Isolated human Purkinje cell from a 53-year-old male (phase contrast, × 700).

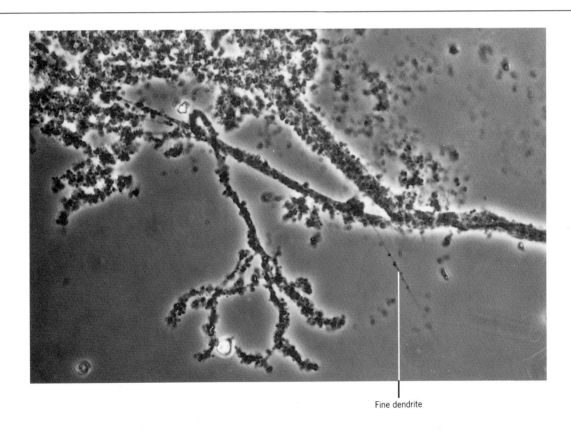

Fine dendrite

Figure 241   Teased dendrites from the human Purkinje cell of the previous specimen (phase contrast, × 700).

Fine granules adhere to the dendrites.

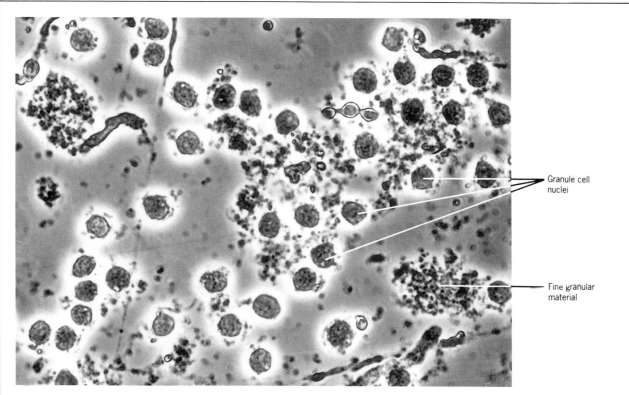

Granule cell
nuclei

Fine granular
material

Figure 242 Isolated human cerebellar granule cells and fine granular material from a 55-year-old male (phase contrast, × 700). It is difficult to see cytoplasm around these cells.

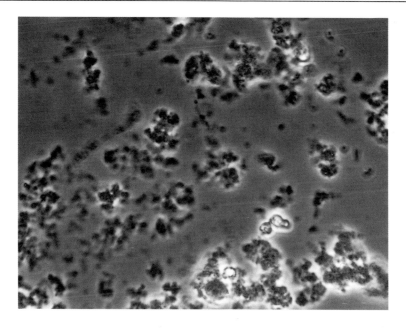

Figure 243 Isolated fine granular material of human cerebellar grey matter from an 80-year-old female (phase contrast, × 700).

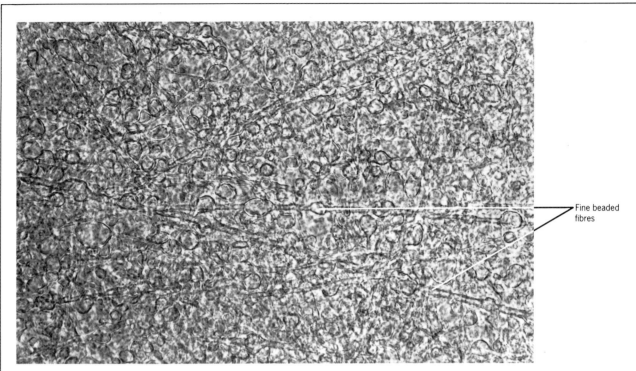

Fine beaded fibres

Figure 244   Thin slab of human cerebellar white matter from the centre of a folium from a 71-year-old male, to show fine beaded fibres (phase contrast, × 700).

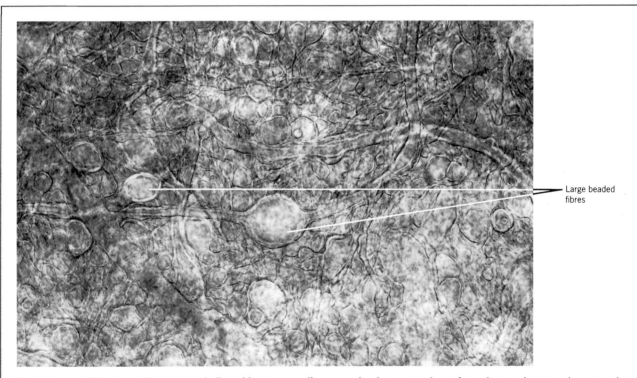

Large beaded fibres

Figure 245   Thin slab of human cerebellar white matter adjacent to the dentate nucleus, from the previous specimen, to show large beaded fibres and droplets (phase contrast, × 700).

There is a large variation in fibre diameters between the fibres seen in this and the previous figure.

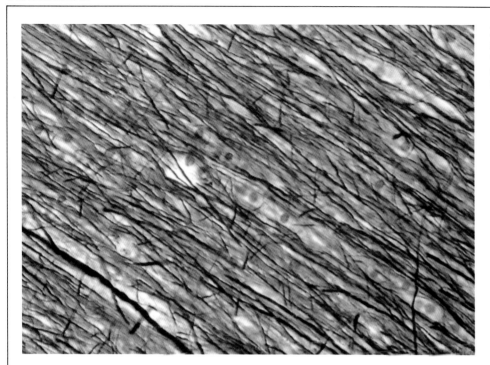

Figure 246 Section of human cerebellar white matter, stained with Palmgren's stain, to show a tract of fine fibres (bright field, × 610).

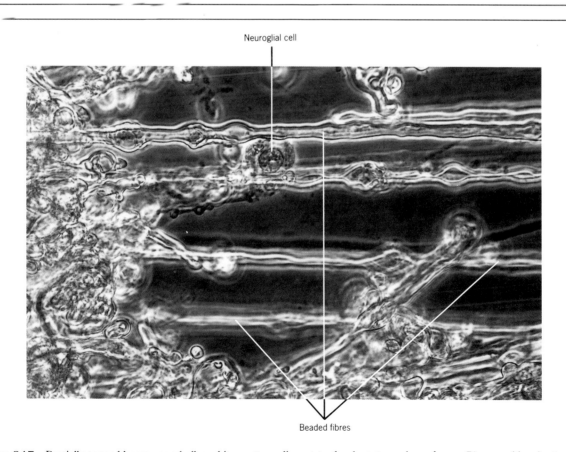

Neuroglial cell

Beaded fibres

Figure 247 Partially teased human cerebellar white matter adjacent to the dentate nucleus, from a 71-year-old male, to show beaded fibres and neuroglial cells (phase contrast, × 700).

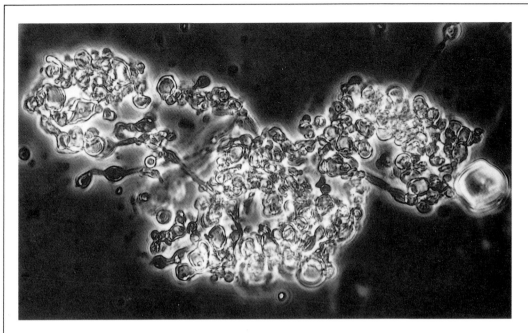

Figure 248   Teased human cerebellar white matter from an 80-year-old female, to show beaded fibres and droplets (phase contrast, × 800).

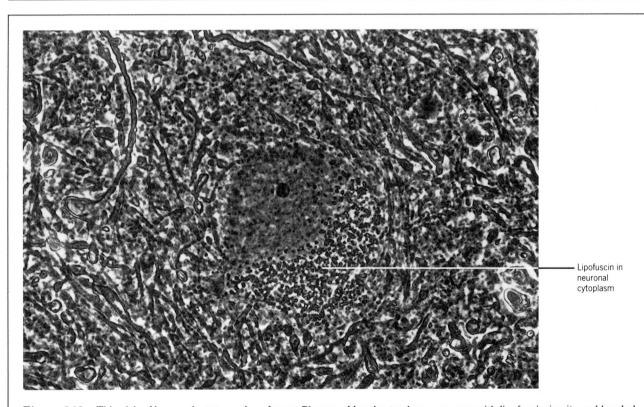

Lipofuscin in neuronal cytoplasm

Figure 249   Thin slab of human dentate nucleus from a 71-year-old male, to show a neuron with lipofuscin *in situ* and beaded fibres (phase contrast, × 700).

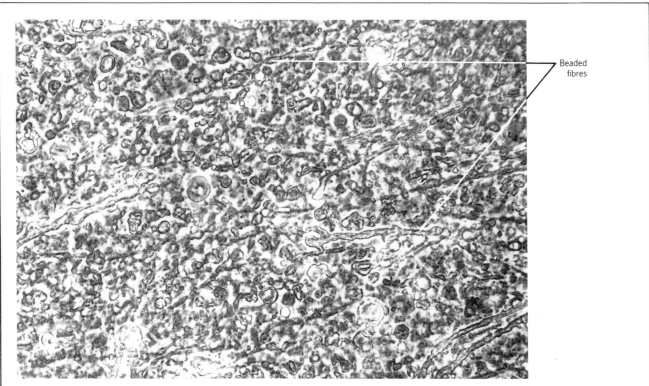

Beaded
fibres

Figure 250 Thin slab of human dentate nucleus from the previous specimen, to show beaded fibres and droplets (phase contrast, × 700).

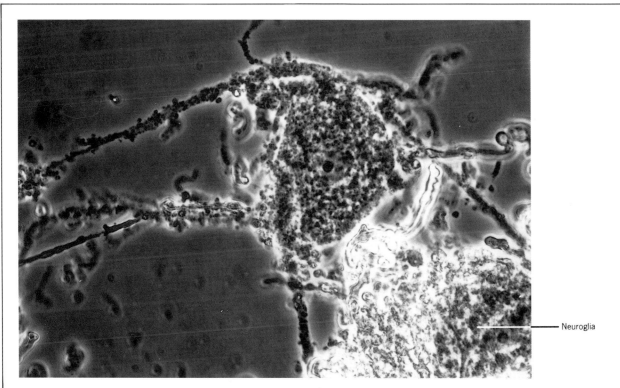

Neuroglia

Figure 251 Isolated guinea-pig neuron with associated neuroglia from the dentate nucleus (phase contrast, × 700).

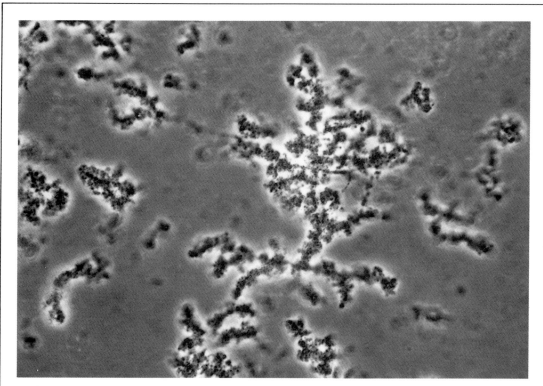

Figure 252 Teased neuroglia from the rabbit dentate nucleus, to show fine granular material (phase contrast, × 700).

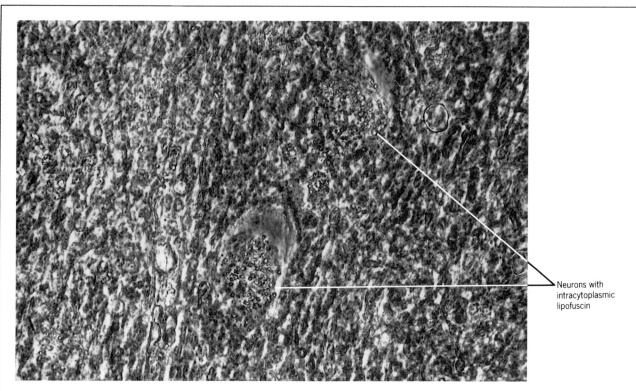

Neurons with intracytoplasmic lipofuscin

Figure 253 Thin slab of human fastigial nucleus from a 71-year-old male, to show neurons *in situ* with associated lipofuscin (phase contrast, × 700).

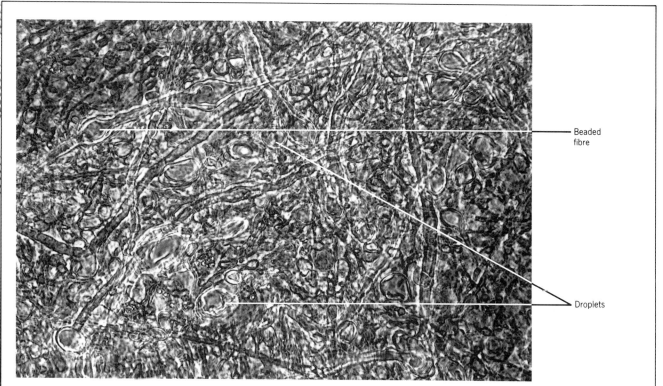

Beaded
fibre

Droplets

Figure 254 Thin slab of human white matter adjacent to the fastigial nucleus, from the previous specimen, to show beaded fibres and droplets (phase contrast, × 700).

SECTION
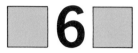
6

SPINAL CORD AND GANGLIA

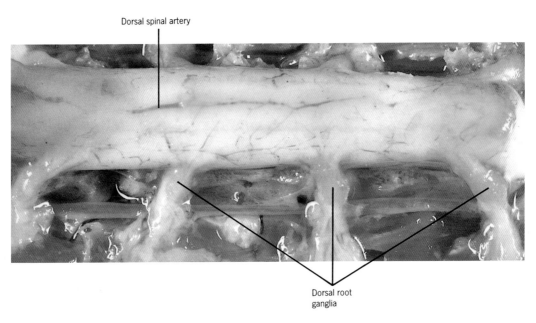

Figure 255 Dissection of rat spinal cord to show the position of dorsal root ganglia (× 6).

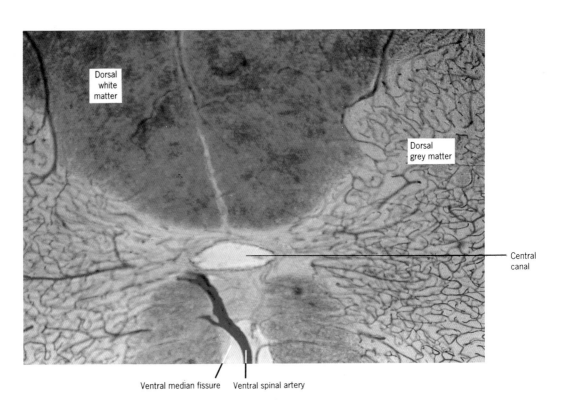

Figure 256 Section of injected cat spinal cord to show that there are more blood vessels in the grey than the white matter (× 60).

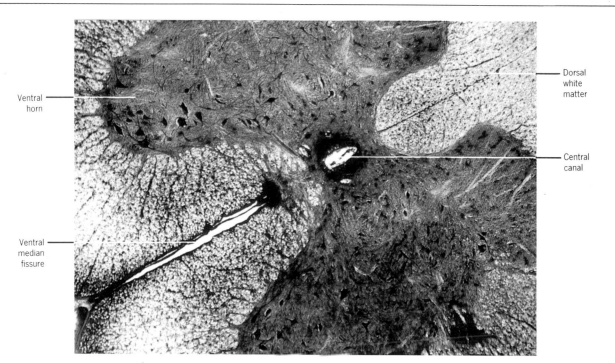

Ventral horn

Dorsal white matter

Central canal

Ventral median fissure

Figure 257 Section of cat spinal cord stained with a silver stain to show the distribution of black-staining ventral horn cells in the grey matter (bright field, × 40).

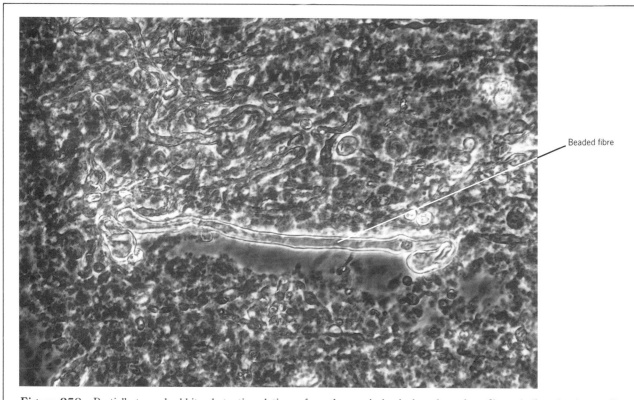

Beaded fibre

Figure 258 Partially teased rabbit substantia gelatinosa from the cervical spinal cord, to show fibres, believed to be myelinated (phase contrast, × 700).

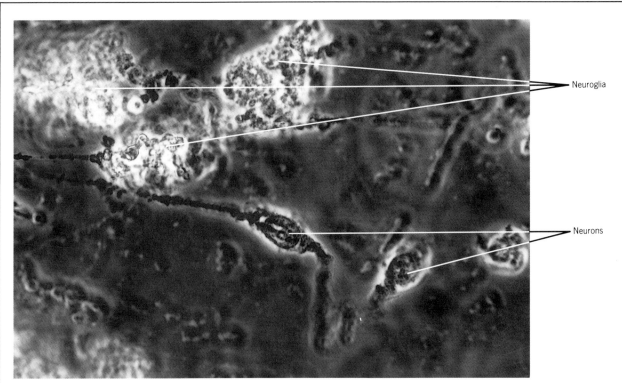

Figure 259   Teased rabbit substantia gelatinosa from the cervical spinal cord, to show bipolar neurons and associated neuroglia (phase contrast, × 700).

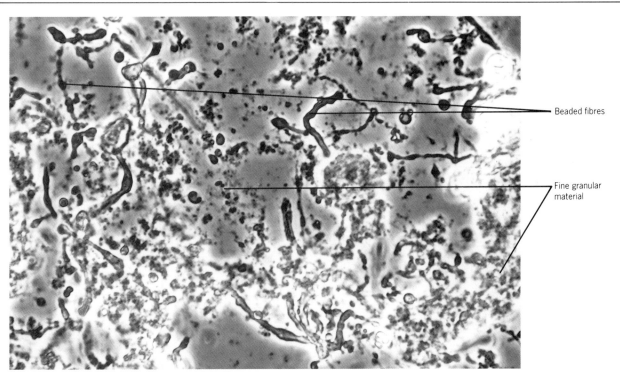

Figure 260   Teased guinea-pig substantia gelatinosa from the cervical spinal cord, to show a small neuron, beaded fibres and fine granular material (phase contrast, × 700).

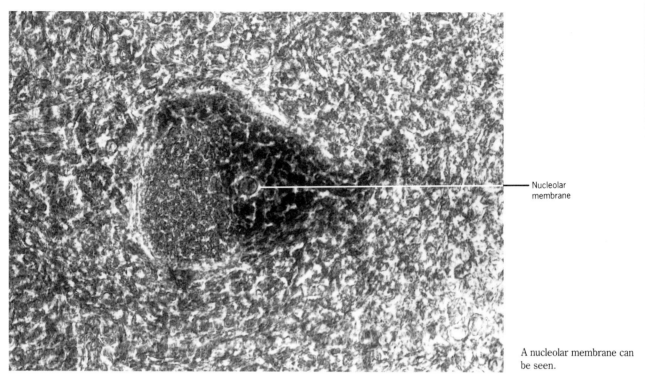

Nucleolar
membrane

A nucleolar membrane can
be seen.

Figure 261   Thin slab of human anterior horn from the cervical spinal cord from an 89-year-old female, to show anterior horn cell *in situ* (phase contrast, × 700).

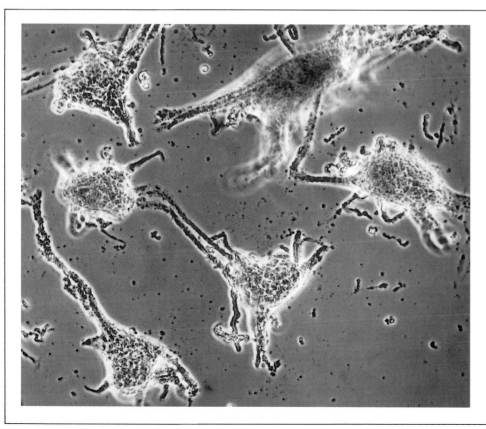

Figure 262   Isolated rabbit ventral horn cells from the cervical spinal cord (phase contrast, × 335).

The term 'neuron' was coined by Waldeyer-Hartz in 1891.

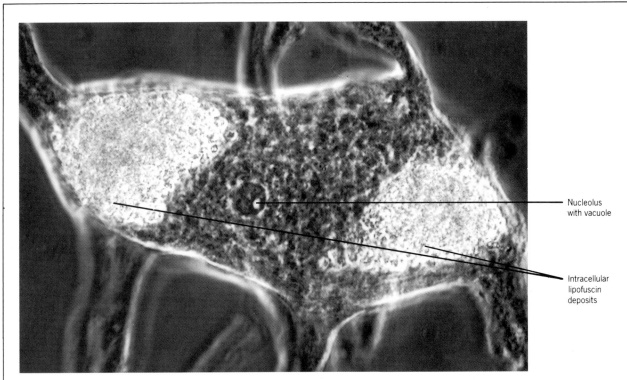

Nucleolus
with vacuole

Intracellular
lipofuscin
deposits

Figure 263 Isolated human anterior horn cell from the cervical spinal cord of a 75-year-old male, to show the large intracellular lipofuscin deposits, the nucleus and the nucleolus (phase contrast, × 1100).

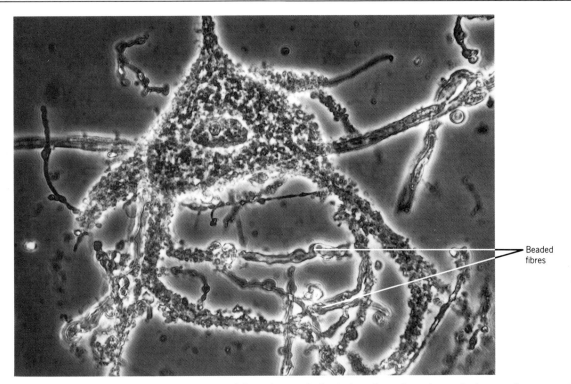

Beaded
fibres

Figure 264 Isolated rabbit anterior horn cell from the cervical spinal cord, to show the nucleolar membrane, small and medium size beaded fibres, and a capillary (phase contrast, × 700).

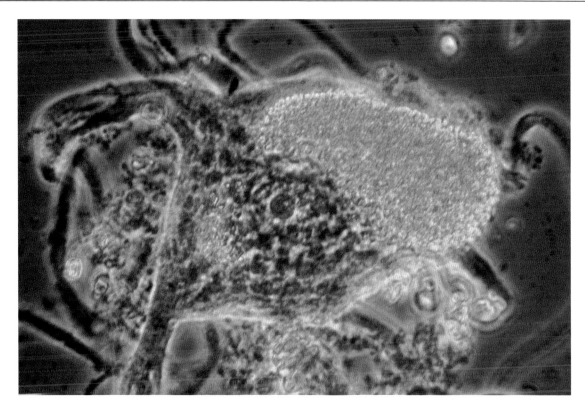

Figure 265   Isolated human anterior horn cell from a 74-year-old male (phase contrast, × 720).

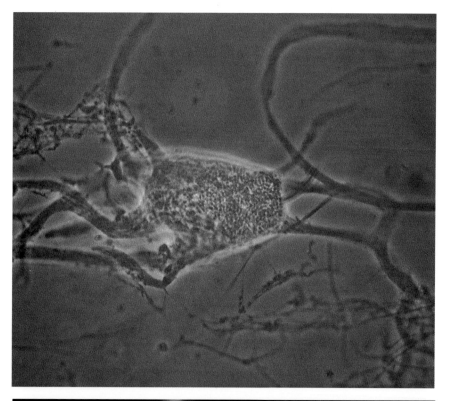

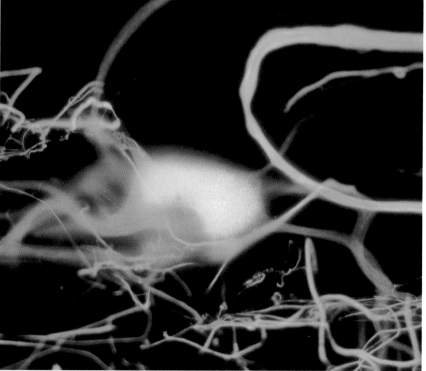

Figure 266   İsolated human anterior horn cell of an 82-year-old male, stained with anti-neurofilament 200 kD protein, by phase contrast (above) and after excitation with blue light of 450–490 nm (below) (× 500).

As in Figure 221, the lipofuscin fluoresces brightly as do probably unmyelinated fibres, but the main dendrites only weakly.

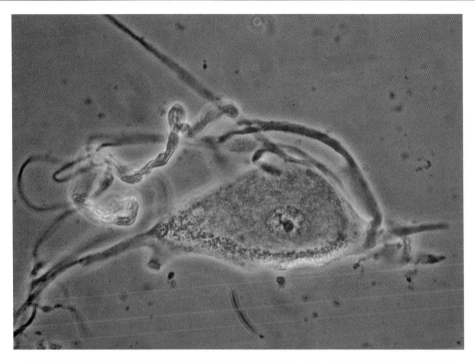

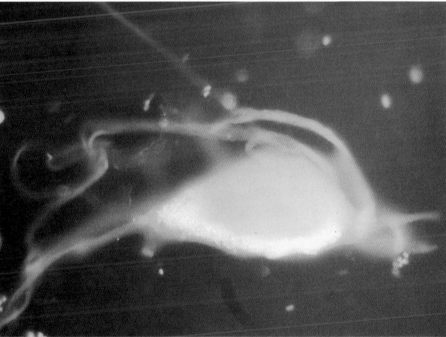

Figure 267   Isolated human anterior horn cell of a 64-year-old male, stained with anti-glial fibrillary acidic protein, by phase contrast (above) and after excitation with blue light of 450–490 nm (below) (× 500).

Compare with the previous figure.

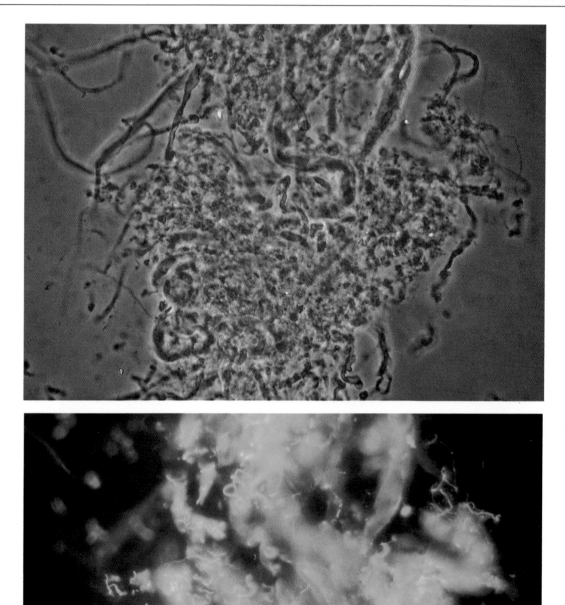

Figure 268   Isolated human neuroglia from the anterior horn of a 64-year-old male, stained with anti-glial fibrillary acidic protein, by phase contrast (above) and after excitation with blue light of 450–490 nm (below) (× 500).

Short fine fibres are fluorescing brightly. Compare with the fibres in Figure 226.

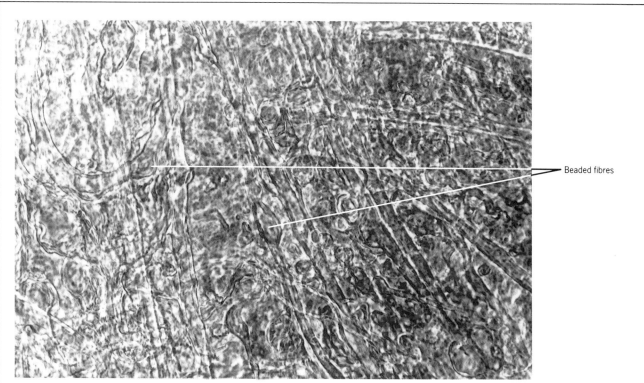

Beaded fibres

Figure 269 Thin slab of human gracile tract from the cervical spinal cord of an 89-year-old female, to show beaded fibres *in situ* (phase contrast, × 700).

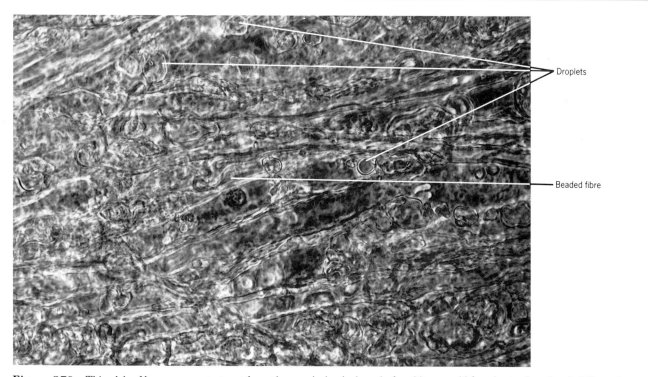

Droplets

Beaded fibre

Figure 270 Thin slab of human cuneate tract from the cervical spinal cord of an 89-year-old female, to show beaded fibres *in situ* and droplets (phase contrast, × 700).

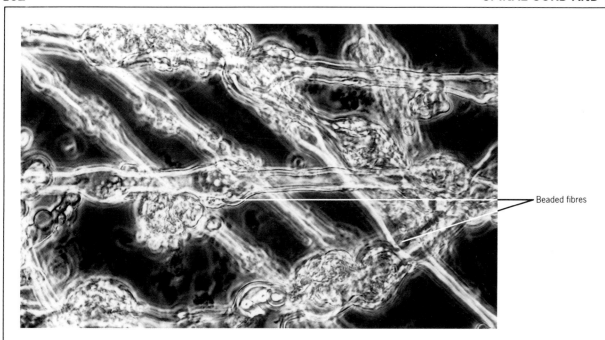

Figure 271   Teased human cuneate tract from the previous specimen, to show beaded fibres (phase contrast, × 700).

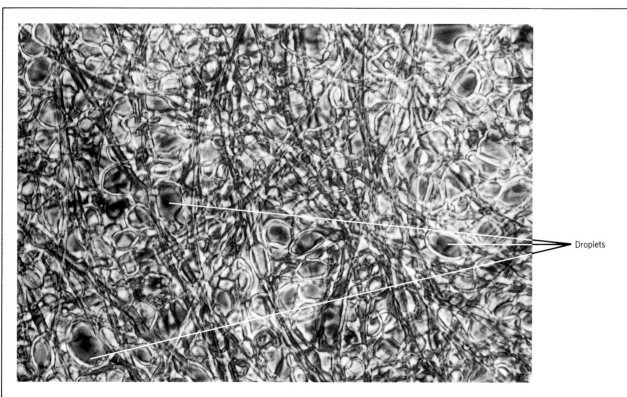

Figure 272   Thin slab of fresh rat dorsal region of cervical spinal cord, to show beaded fibres and droplets (phase contrast, × 700).

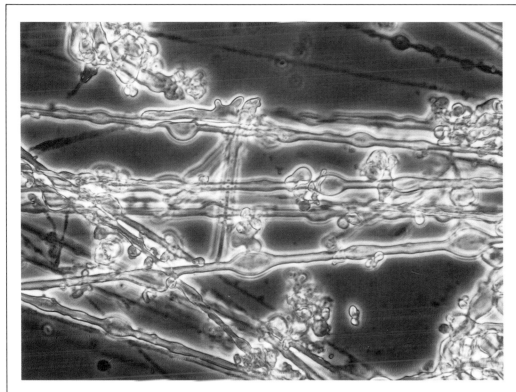

Figure 273 Teased fresh rat beaded fibres from the dorsal cervical spinal cord (phase contrast, × 700).

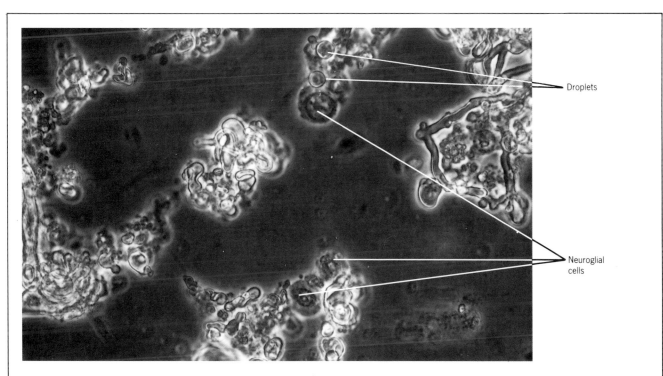

Figure 274 Teased fresh guinea-pig dorsal white matter from the sacral spinal cord, to show droplets and neuroglial cells (phase contrast, × 700).

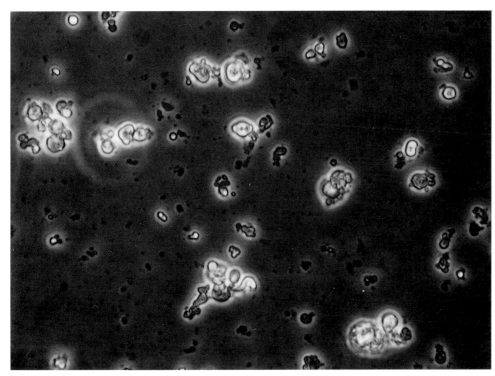

Figure 275 Teased freshly killed rabbit dorsal white matter from the cervical spinal cord, to show isolated droplets (phase contrast, × 700).

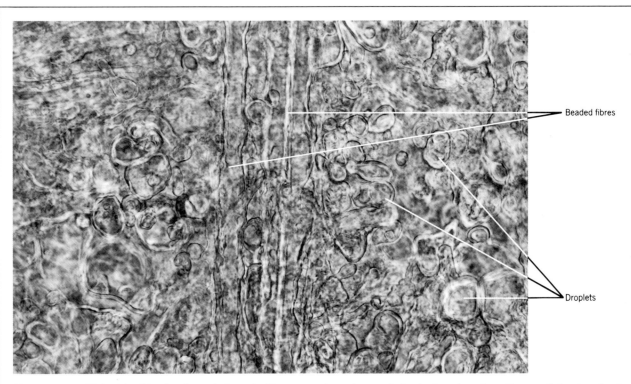

Figure 276 Thin slab of fresh guinea-pig lateral white matter from the cervical spinal cord to show fibres and droplets *in situ* (phase contrast, × 700).

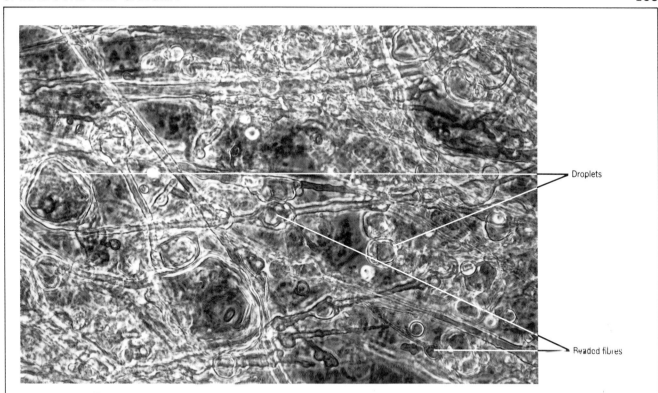

Droplets

Beaded fibres

Figure 277 Partially teased human vestibulospinal tract from the cervical spinal cord of an 89-year-old female, to show beaded fibres and droplets (phase contrast, × 700).

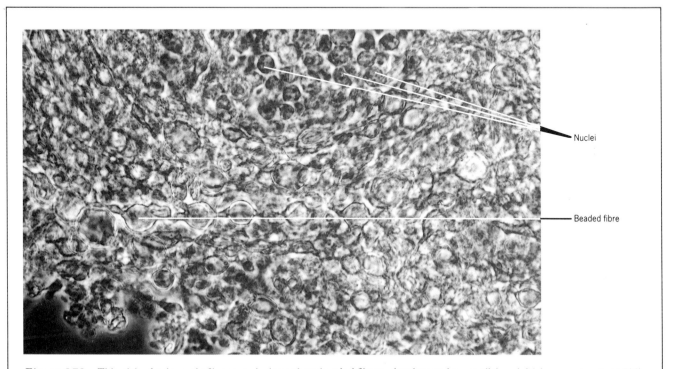

Nuclei

Beaded fibre

Figure 278 Thin slab of guinea-pig filum terminale to show beaded fibres, droplets and neuroglial nuclei (phase contrast, × 700).

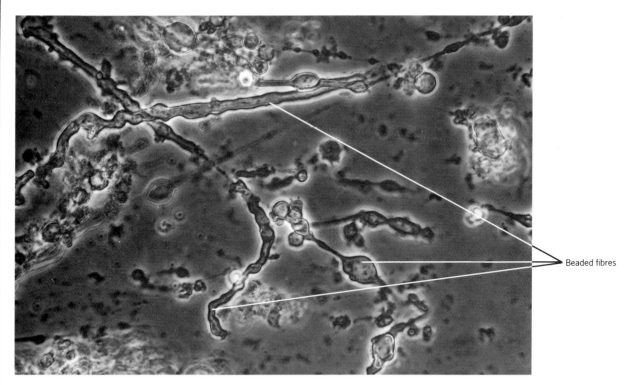

Figure 279   Teased fresh guinea-pig filum terminale to show beaded fibres (phase contrast, × 700).

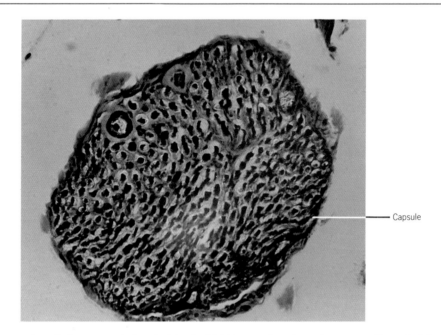

Figure 280   Transverse section of a human ventral root stained with Palmgren's stain to show nerve fibres (bright field, × 610).

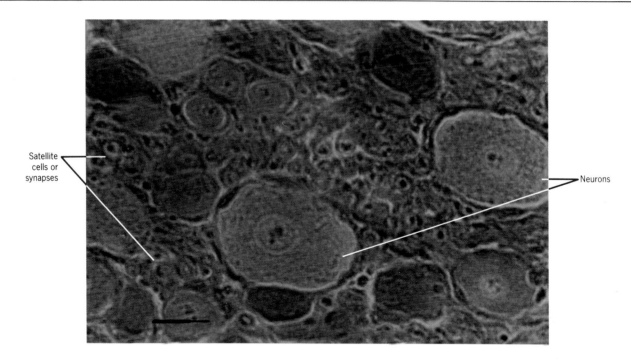

Satellite cells or synapses

Neurons

Figure 281   Section of a human dorsal root ganglion stained with haematoxylin and eosin (bright field, × 610).

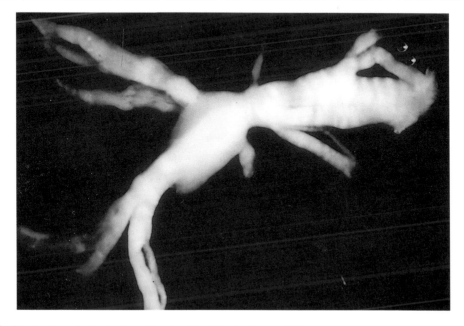

Figure 282   Isolated rat cervical spinal ganglion (vertical illumination, × 20).

Satellite cells or synapses

Ganglion
cell

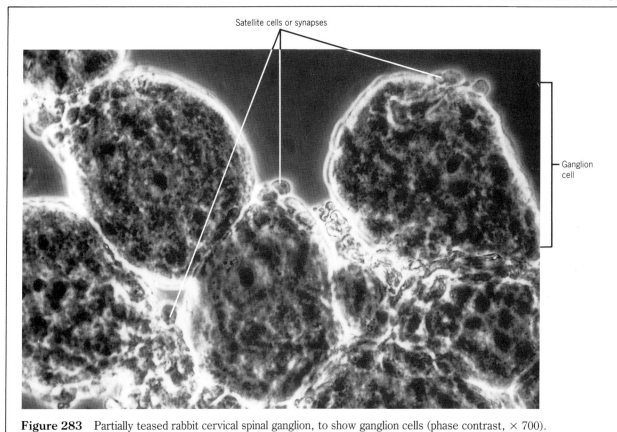

Figure 283   Partially teased rabbit cervical spinal ganglion, to show ganglion cells (phase contrast, × 700).

Dendrite

Figure 284   Isolated rat ganglion cell from cervical spinal ganglion (phase contrast, × 800).

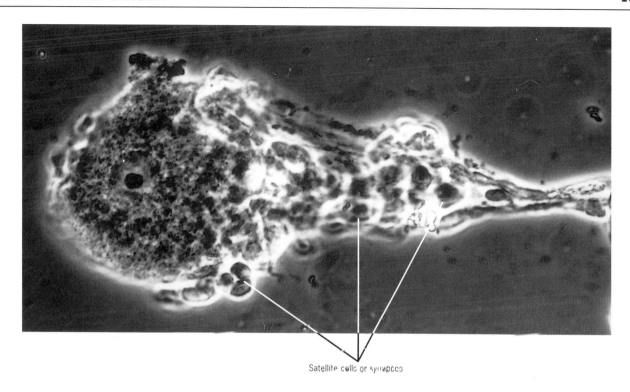

Satellite cells or synapses

Figure 285 Isolated rabbit ganglion cell from cervical spinal ganglion to show associated 'satellite' cells or synapses (phase contrast, × 800).

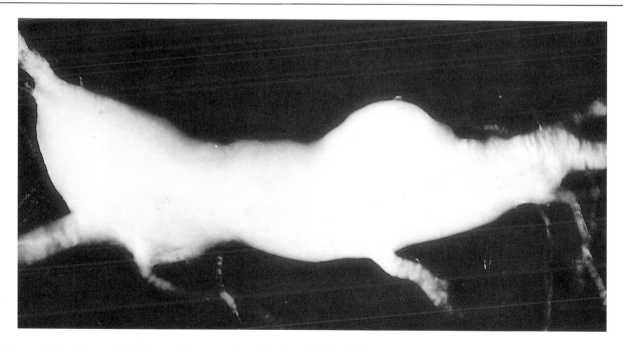

Figure 286 Dissected rabbit superior cervical ganglion (vertical illumination, × 20).

This ganglion is sympathetic.

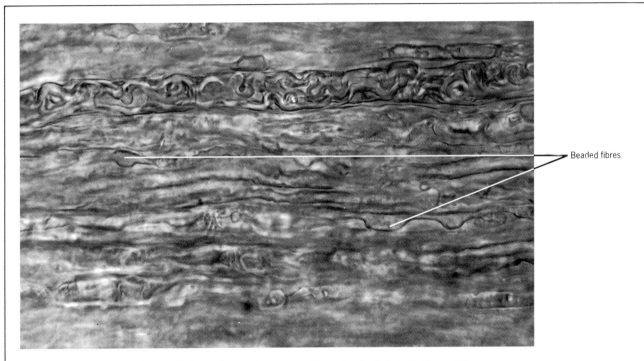

Beaded fibres

Figure 287   Rat superior cervical ganglion to show nerve fibres *in situ* (bright field, × 800).

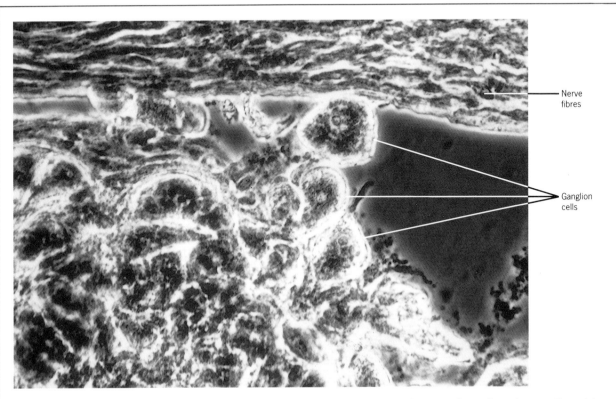

Nerve fibres

Ganglion cells

Figure 288   Partially teased superior cervical ganglion from 4-week-old rat, to show ganglion cells and nerve fibres (phase contrast, × 700).

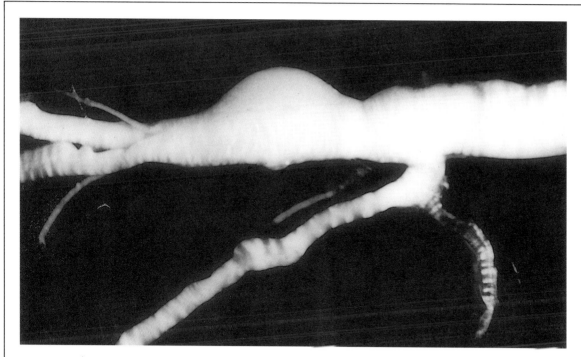

Figure 289 Dissected rabbit vagal ganglion (vertical illumination, × 20).

This ganglion is parasympathetic.

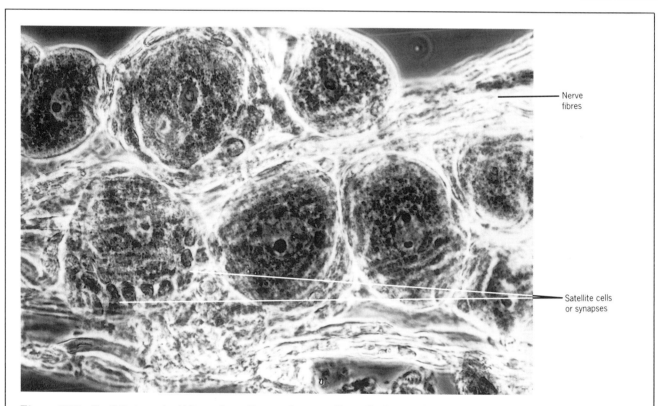

Figure 290 Partially teased rabbit vagal ganglion, to show ganglion cells, 'satellite' cells or synapses, and nerve fibres (phase contrast, × 700).

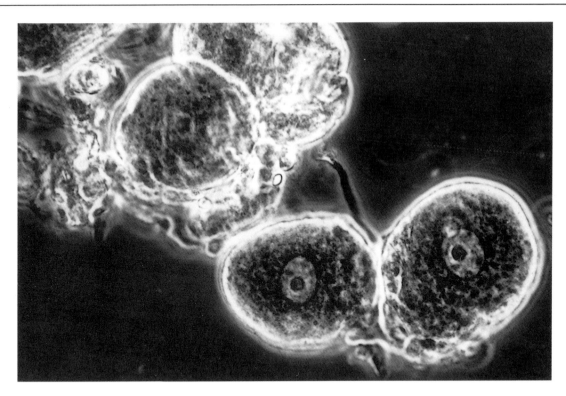

Figure 291   Teased rabbit ganglion cells from the previous specimen (phase contrast, × 800).

Note the low refractive index of the nucleoplasm.

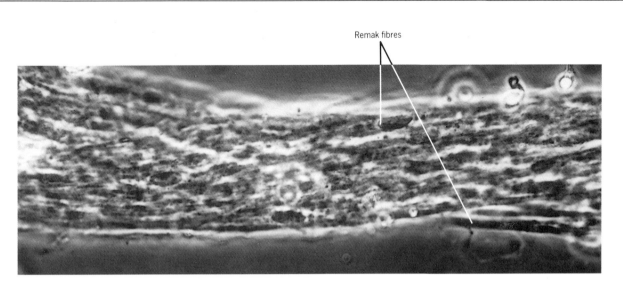

Figure 292   Partially teased mouse sympathetic nerve to the ileum, to show Remak fibres *in situ* (phase contrast, × 800).

These fibres were described by Remak in 1836.

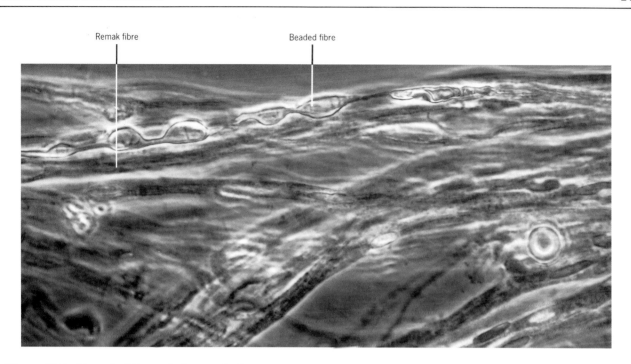

Figure 293   Teased rabbit cervical sympathetic nerve, to show a beaded fibre and Remak fibres (phase contrast, × 800).

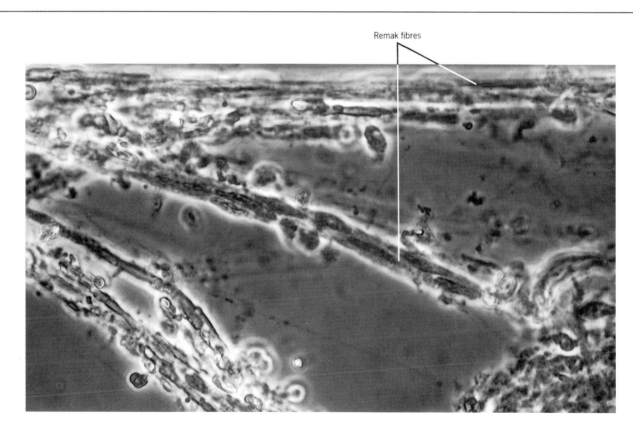

Figure 294   Teased guinea-pig cervical sympathetic nerve, to show Remak fibres (phase contrast, × 800).

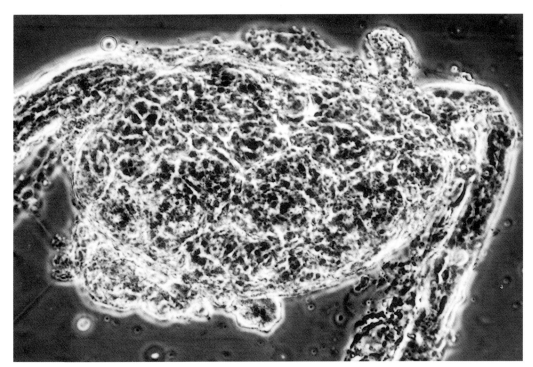

Figure 295   Isolated mouse sublingual ganglion, to show ganglion cells *in situ* (bright field, × 500).

This ganglion is parasympathetic.

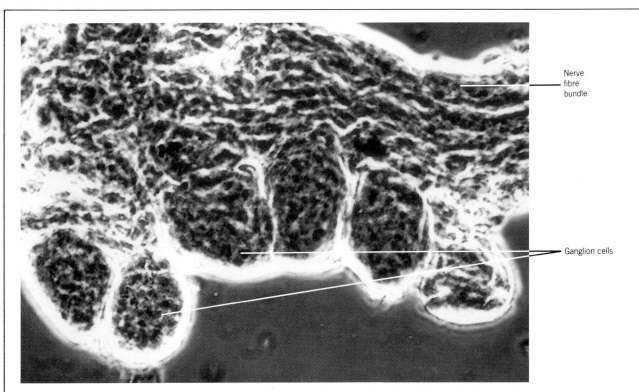

Nerve
fibre
bundle

Ganglion cells

Figure 296   Partially teased mouse sublingual ganglion, to show ganglion cells and associated nerve fibres (phase contrast, × 1100).

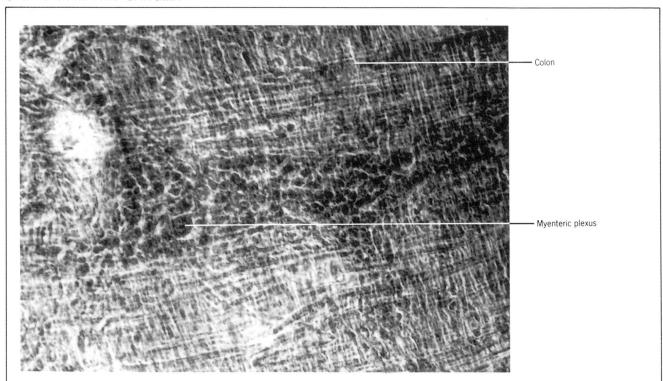

Figure 297 Myenteric plexus in guinea-pig colon *in situ* (bright field, × 270).

This plexus is parasympathetic.

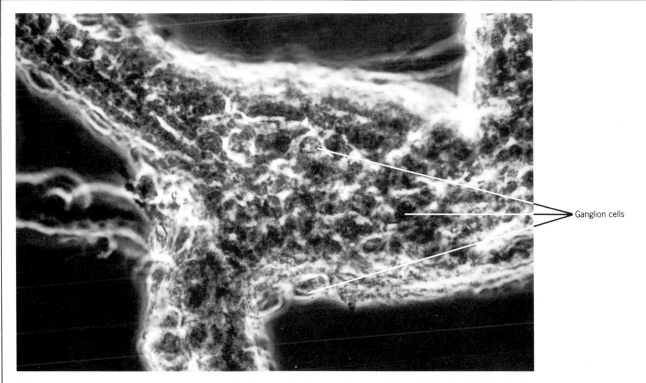

Figure 298 Dissected guinea-pig myenteric plexus of colon, to show ganglion cells *in situ* (bright field, × 700).

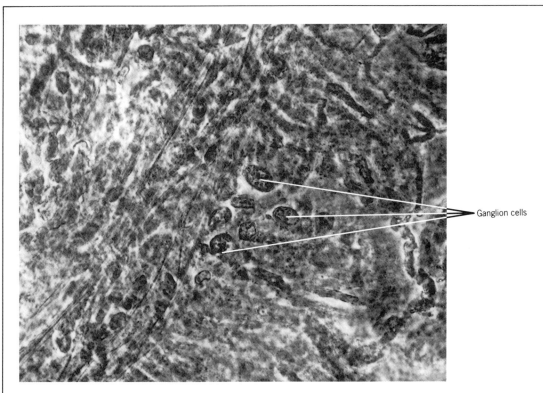

Figure 299   Guinea-pig myenteric plexus of colon *in situ*, to show ganglion cells (bright field, × 700).

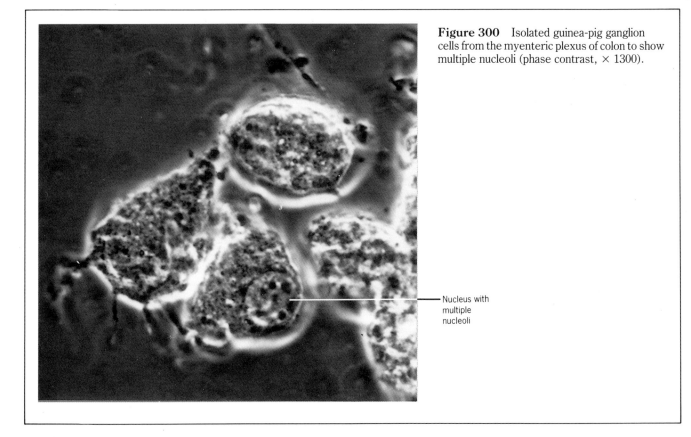

Figure 300   Isolated guinea-pig ganglion cells from the myenteric plexus of colon to show multiple nucleoli (phase contrast, × 1300).

SECTION
7

CRANIAL NERVES AND RETINA

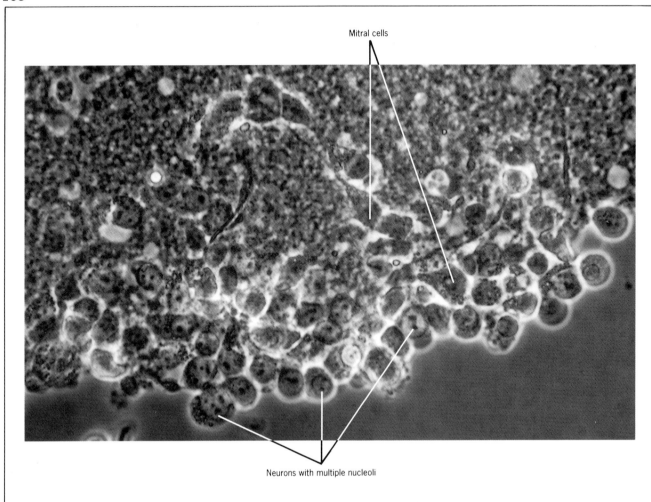

Mitral cells

Neurons with multiple nucleoli

Figure 301 Partially teased rabbit olfactory bulb to show different cell types (phase contrast, × 800).

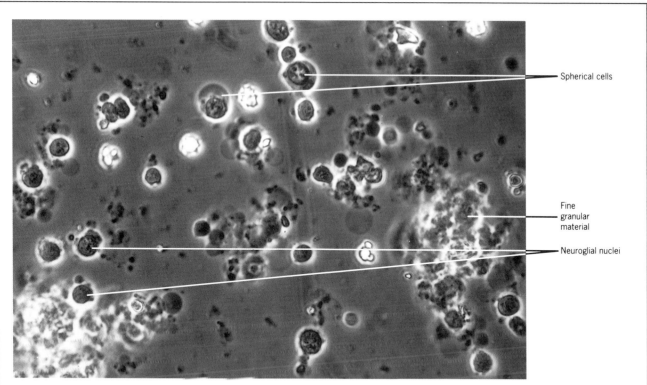

Figure 302 Teased human olfactory bulb from a 75-year-old male, to show spherical cells (phase contrast, × 700).

These are probably neuroglia.

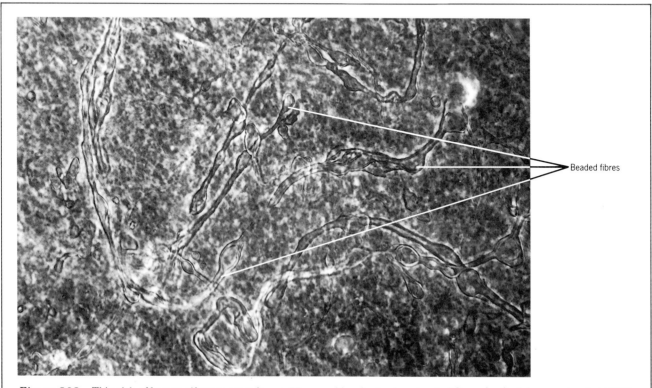

Figure 303 Thin slab of human olfactory tract from a 55-year-old male, to show beaded fibres *in situ* (phase contrast, × 700).

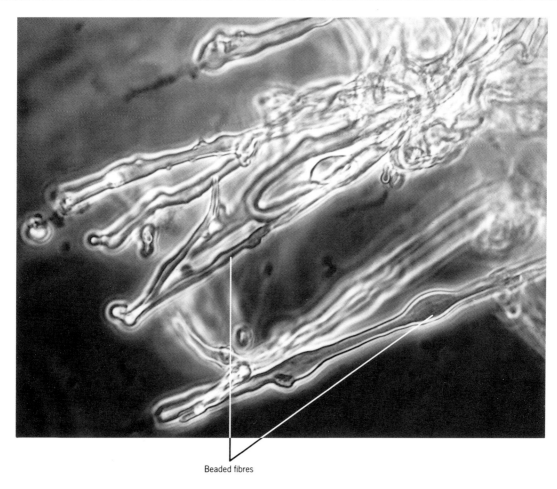

Beaded fibres

Figure 304   Partially teased human olfactory tract from a 75-year-old male, to show fibres (phase contrast, × 1200).

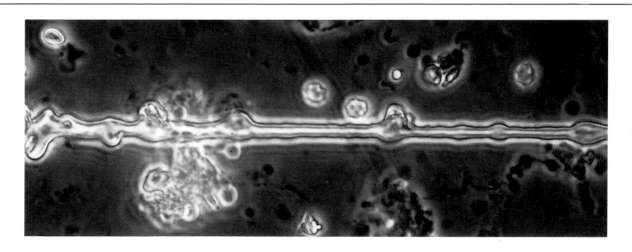

Figure 305   Isolated beaded fibre from the previous specimen (phase contrast, × 800)

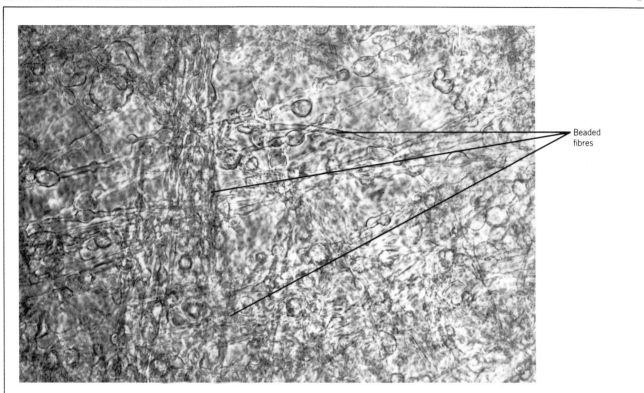

Beaded
fibres

Figure 306   Thin slab of human optic nerve from an 85-year-old female, to show beaded fibres *in situ* (phase contrast, × 700).

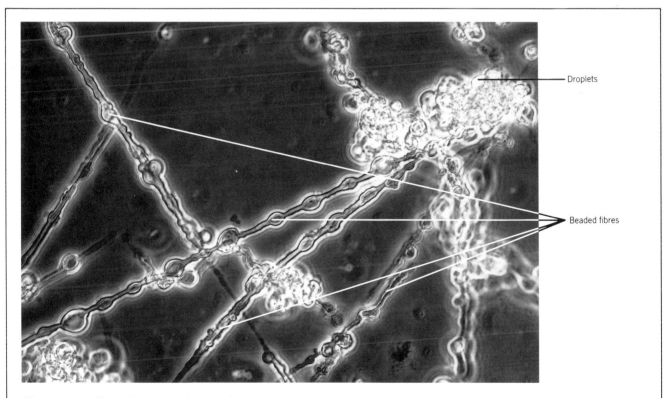

Droplets

Beaded fibres

Figure 307   Teased human optic nerve from an 87-year-old female, to show beaded fibres (phase contrast, × 700).

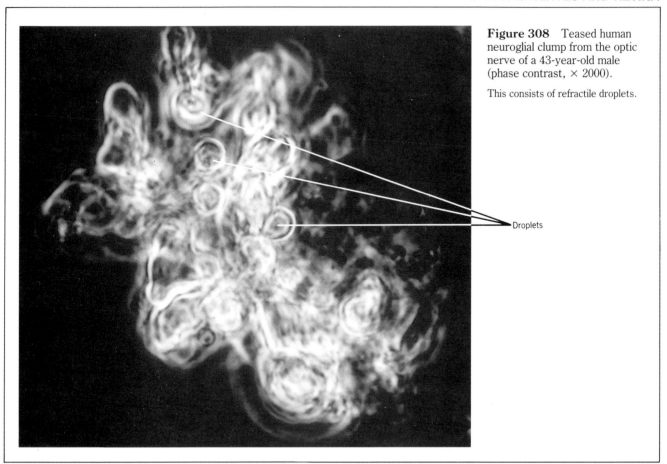

Figure 308 Teased human neuroglial clump from the optic nerve of a 43-year-old male (phase contrast, × 2000).

This consists of refractile droplets.

Droplets

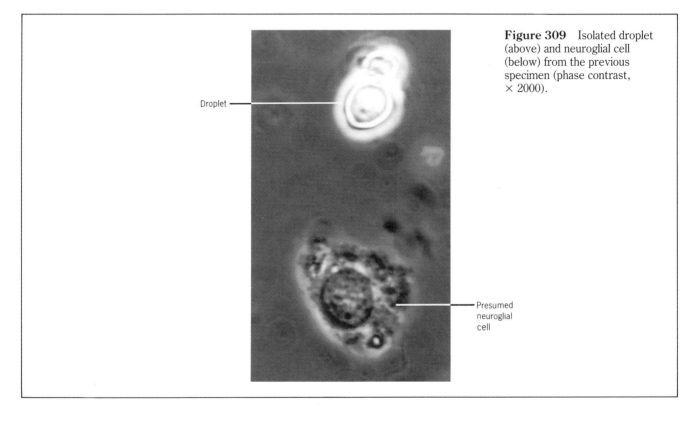

Figure 309 Isolated droplet (above) and neuroglial cell (below) from the previous specimen (phase contrast, × 2000).

Droplet

Presumed neuroglial cell

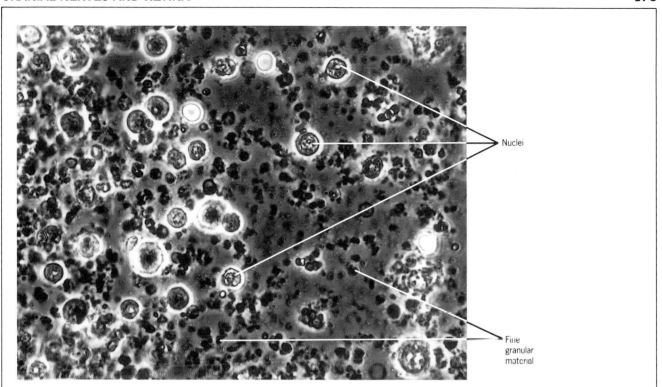

Nuclei

Fine
granular
material

Figure 310 Neuroglial nuclei and fine granular material teased from the optic nerve of a 1-week-old rat (phase contrast, × 700).

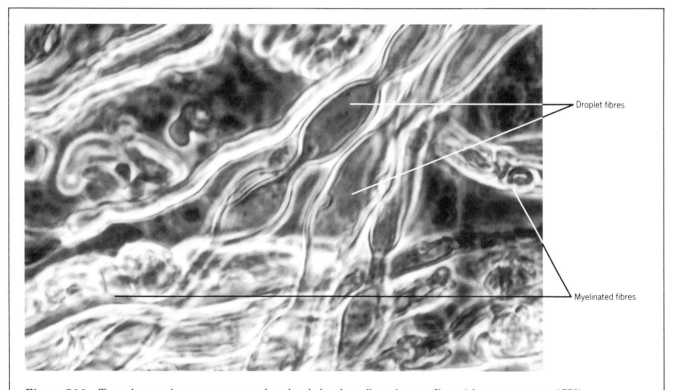

Droplet fibres

Myelinated fibres

Figure 311 Teased rat oculomotor nerve, to show beaded and myelinated nerve fibres (phase contrast, × 1750).

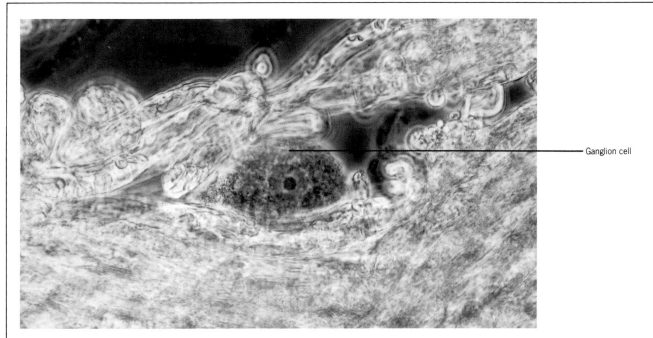

Ganglion cell

Figure 312   Partially teased rat trigeminal nerve to show a ganglion cell and myelinated fibres (phase contrast, × 700).

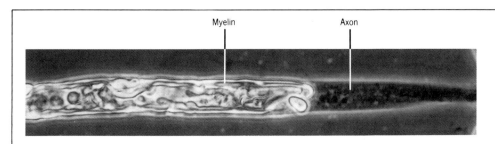

Myelin   Axon

Figure 313   Isolated rabbit myelinated nerve fibre of the abducens nerve, showing the axon from which the sheath has been partly pulled off by teasing (phase contrast, × 700).

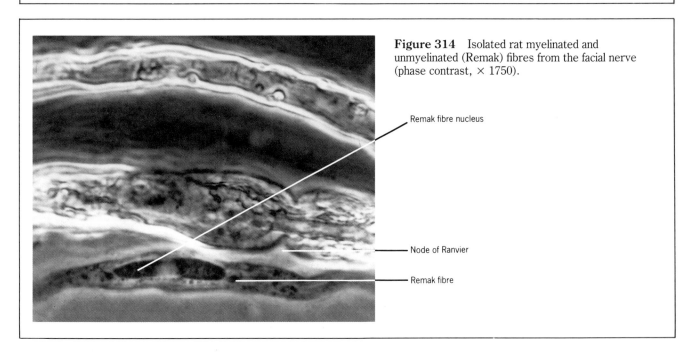

Figure 314   Isolated rat myelinated and unmyelinated (Remak) fibres from the facial nerve (phase contrast, × 1750).

Remak fibre nucleus

Node of Ranvier

Remak fibre

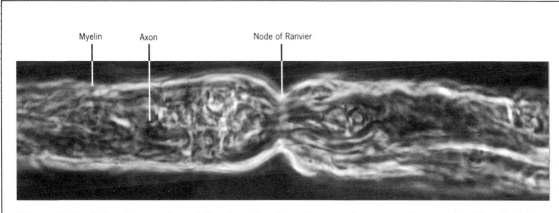

Figure 315 Isolated rat myelinated fibre from the glossopharyngeal nerve, to show a node of Ranvier (phase contrast, × 1750).

Ranvier described them in 1871.

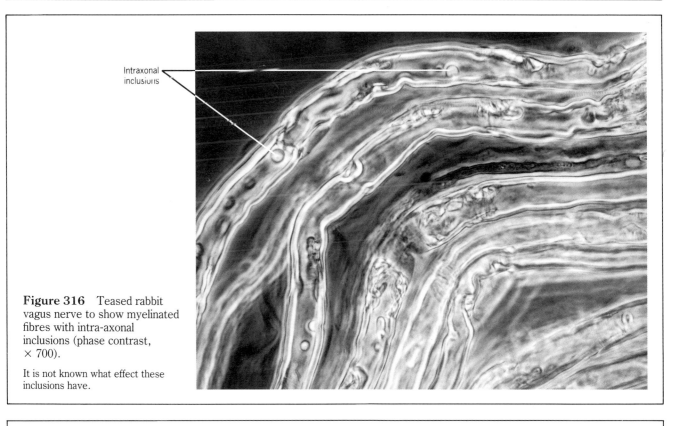

Figure 316 Teased rabbit vagus nerve to show myelinated fibres with intra-axonal inclusions (phase contrast, × 700).

It is not known what effect these inclusions have.

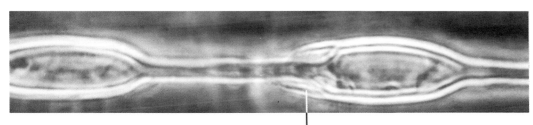

Figure 317 Isolated beaded fibre in rabbit vagus nerve (phase contrast, × 1750).

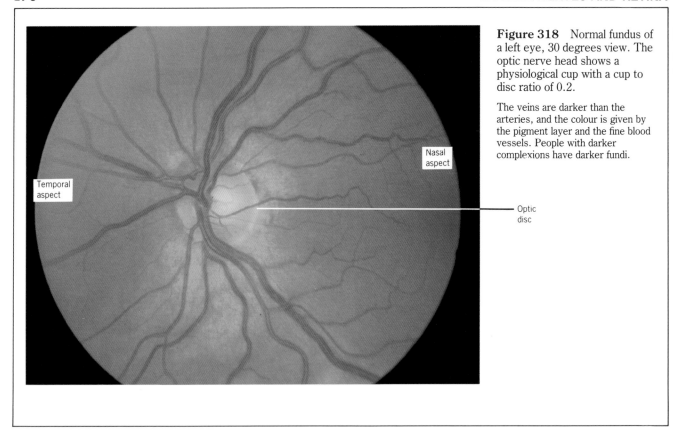

Temporal aspect

Nasal aspect

Optic disc

Figure 318   Normal fundus of a left eye, 30 degrees view. The optic nerve head shows a physiological cup with a cup to disc ratio of 0.2.

The veins are darker than the arteries, and the colour is given by the pigment layer and the fine blood vessels. People with darker complexions have darker fundi.

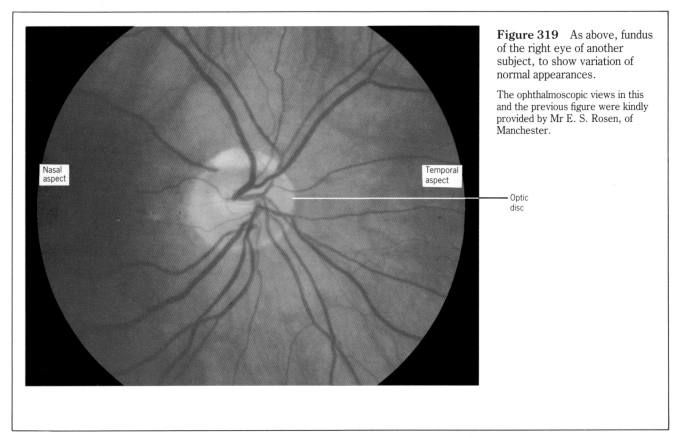

Nasal aspect

Temporal aspect

Optic disc

Figure 319   As above, fundus of the right eye of another subject, to show variation of normal appearances.

The ophthalmoscopic views in this and the previous figure were kindly provided by Mr E. S. Rosen, of Manchester.

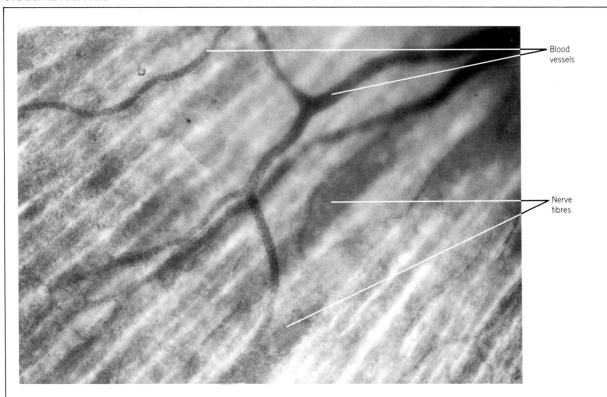

Figure 320   Unteased rabbit retina to show blood vessels and bundles of nerve fibres (bright field, × 85).

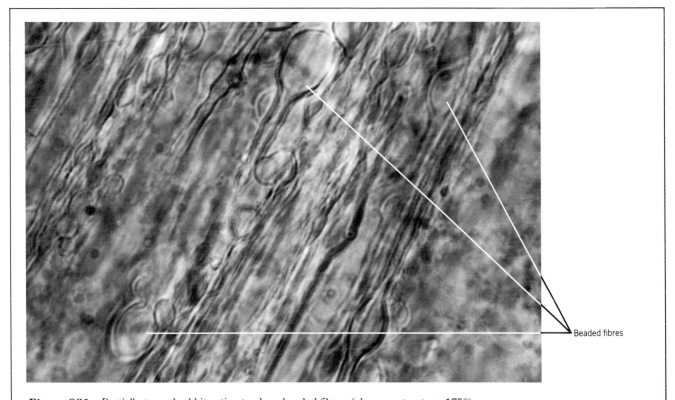

Figure 321   Partially teased rabbit retina to show beaded fibres (phase contrast, × 1750).

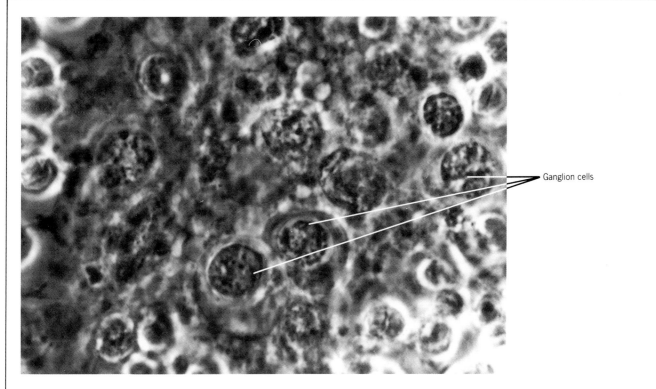

Ganglion cells

Figure 322   Partially teased rabbit retina to show ganglion cells (phase contrast, × 1750).

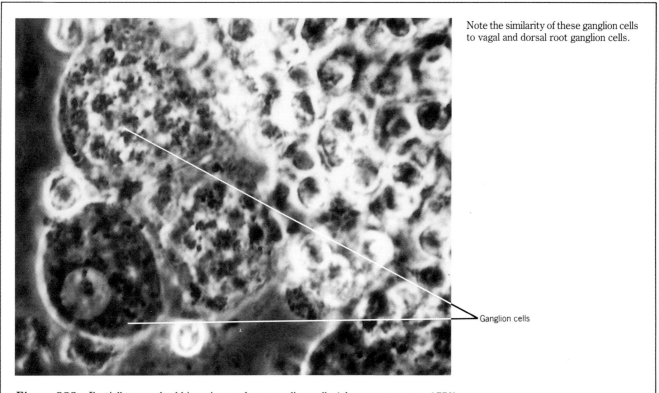

Note the similarity of these ganglion cells to vagal and dorsal root ganglion cells.

Ganglion cells

Figure 323   Partially teased rabbit retina to show ganglion cells (phase contrast, × 1750).

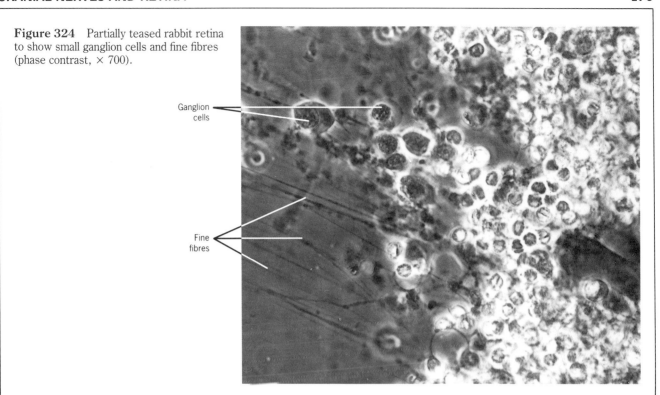

Figure 324 Partially teased rabbit retina to show small ganglion cells and fine fibres (phase contrast, × 700).

Ganglion cells

Fine fibres

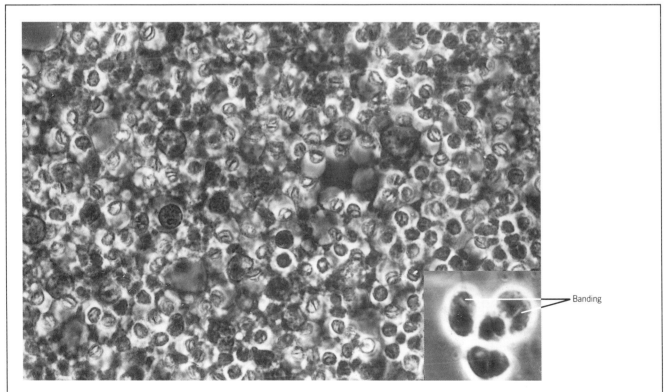

Banding

Figure 325 Partially teased rabbit retina, to show cell bodies of rods and cones (phase contrast, × 700). Inset: rod nuclei (phase contrast, × 1750).

Banding can be seen in rod nuclei.

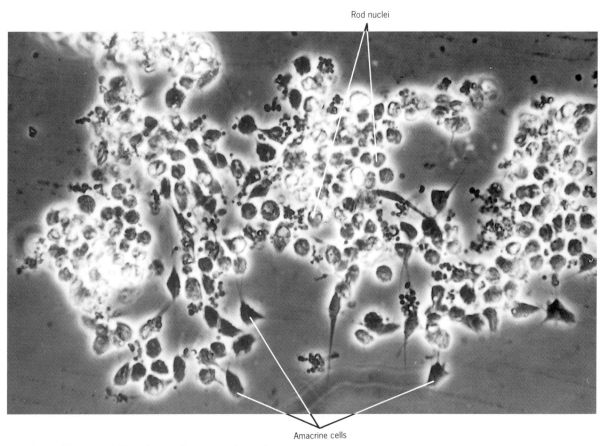

Rod nuclei

Amacrine cells

Figure 326　Teased rabbit retina to show amacrine cells and rod nuclei (phase contrast, × 800).

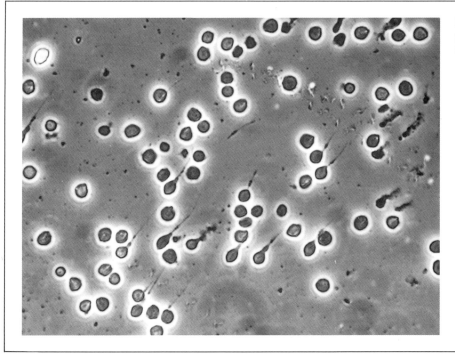

Figure 327　Isolated nuclei, probably of cones, from the central area of rat retina (phase contrast, × 800).

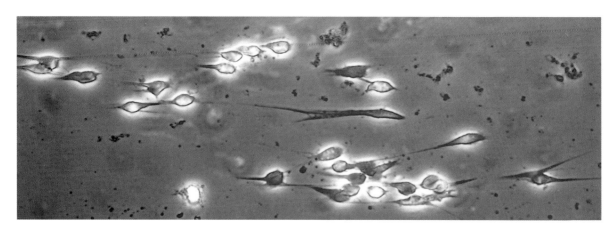

Figure 328 Isolated nuclei, probably of rods, from the central area of rat retina (phase contrast, × 800).

In isolated preparations, it is difficult to differentiate between the nuclei of rods and cones. Their appearances vary between species (Ramon y Cajal, 1892).

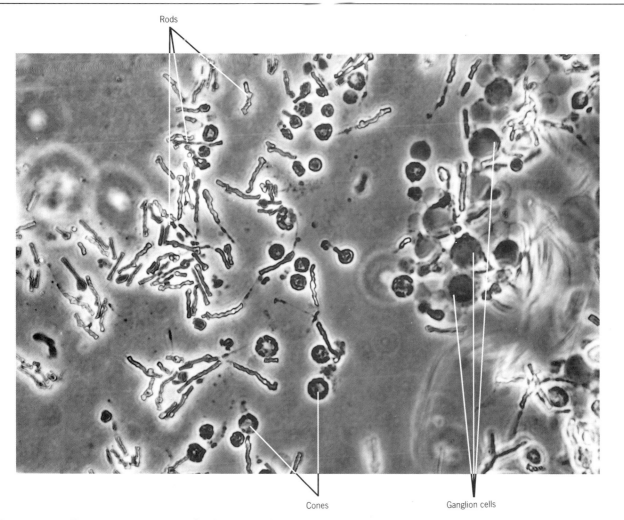

Figure 329 Teased outer segments of rods and ganglion cells from rat retina (phase contrast, × 800).

Pigment cells

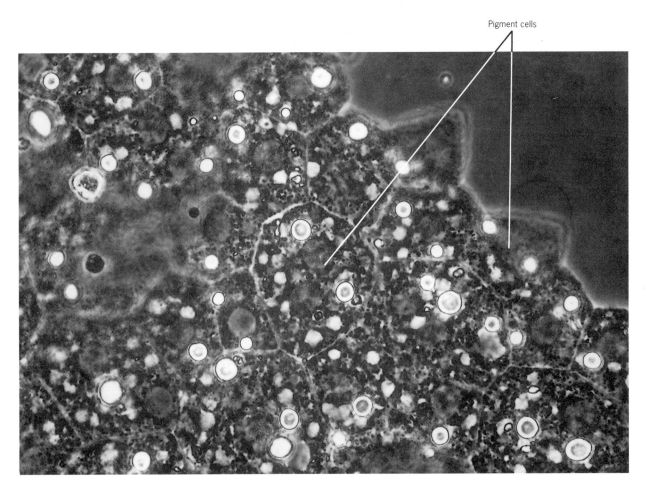

Figure 330 Partially teased rabbit retina to show pigment cell layer (phase contrast, × 800).

SECTION
8

PERIPHERAL NERVES

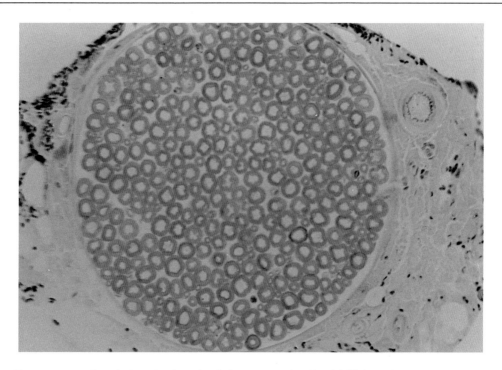

Figure 331   Transverse section of a branch of rabbit sciatic nerve, stained by the Weigert–Pal method, to show the incidence of myelinated fibres (bright field, × 610).

A section of unfixed nerve was first seen by van Leeuwenhoek in 1719.

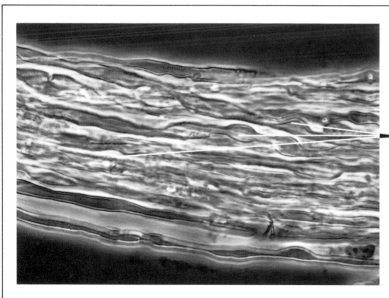

Figure 332 Partially teased 9-day-old mouse phrenic nerve, to show beaded fibres (phase contrast, × 1800).

Myelination was not complete.

Beaded fibres

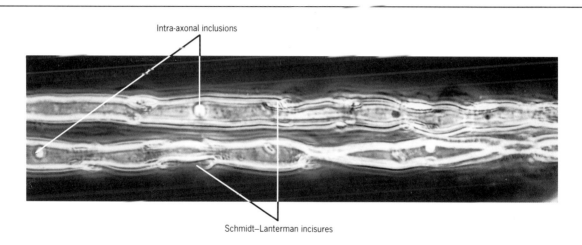

Intra-axonal inclusions

Schmidt–Lanterman incisures

Figure 333 Isolated guinea-pig myelinated nerve fibres from phrenic nerve (phase contrast, × 800).

There are intra-axonal inclusions.

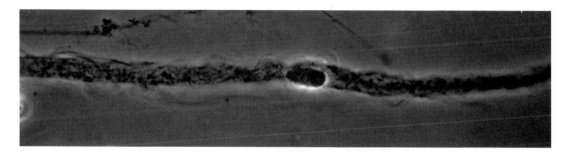

Figure 334 Isolated guinea-pig Remak fibre from phrenic nerve (phase contrast, × 800).

These fibres are rather rare in mixed peripheral nerves.

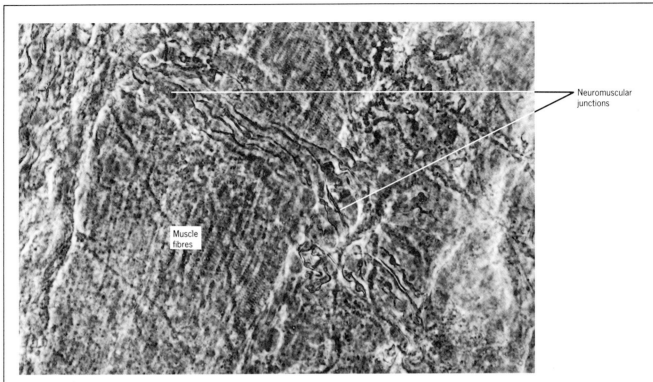

Figure 335 Thin slab of guinea-pig diaphragm including terminations of phrenic nerve, to show neuromuscular junctions (phase contrast, × 700).

Neuromuscular junctions were first seen by Kuhne in 1862.

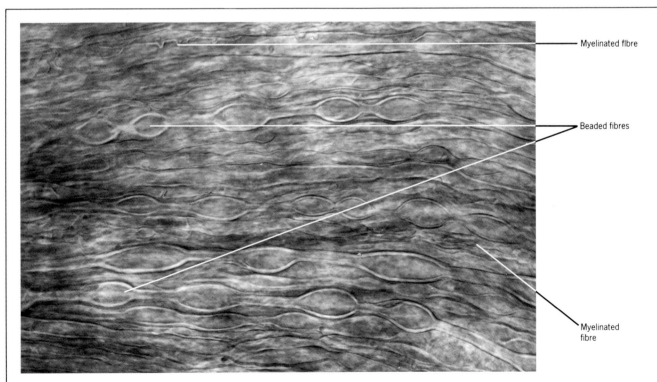

Figure 336 Unteased guinea-pig median nerve, to show beaded and myelinated fibres *in situ* (bright field, × 700).

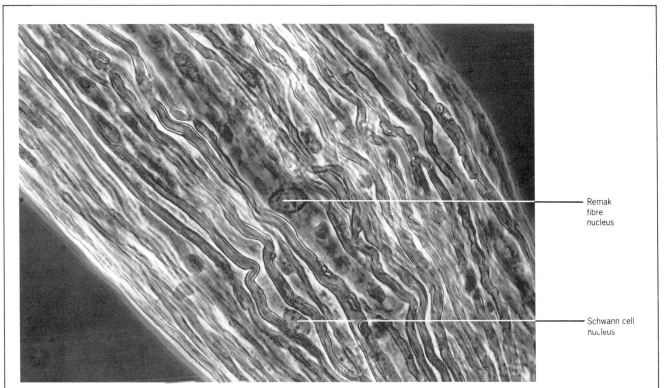

Figure 337 Partially teased 9-day-old mouse median nerve, to show developing myelinated nerve fibres and Schwann cells *in situ* (phase contrast, × 700).

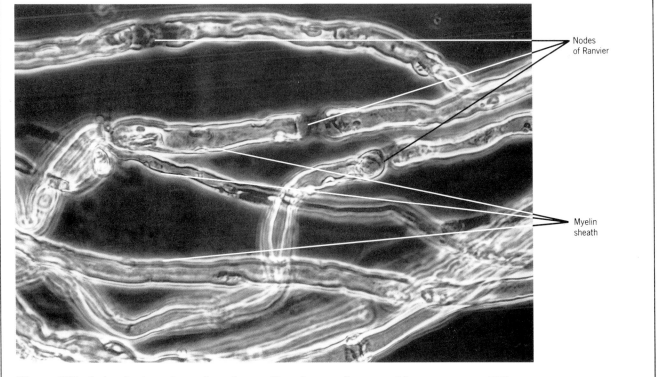

Figure 338 Isolated guinea-pig myelinated nerve fibres from median nerve (phase contrast, × 700).

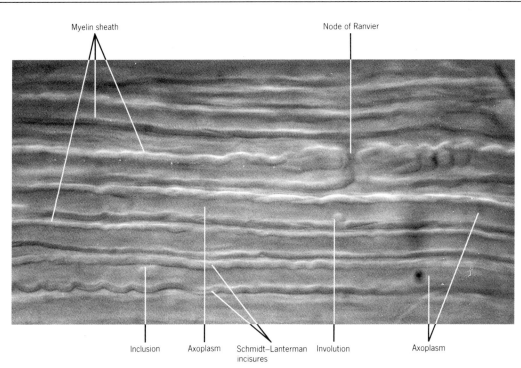

Figure 339   Sciatic nerve of a living mouse *in situ* (incident light, dark ground, × 1000). (By kind permission of Dr S. Hall.)

Note the presence of narrow Schmidt–Lanterman incisures and intra-axonal inclusions (Williams and Hall, 1970).

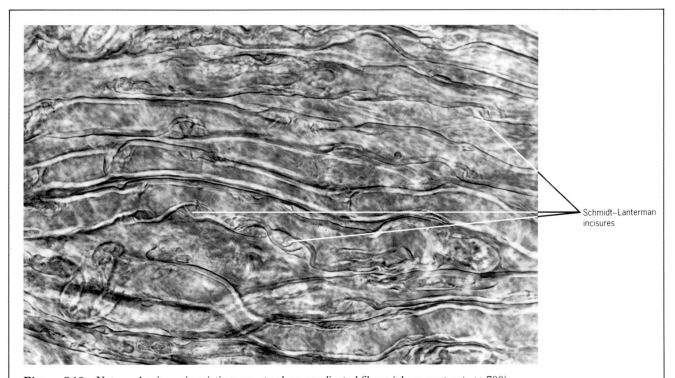

Figure 340   Unteased guinea-pig sciatic nerve, to show myelinated fibres (phase contrast, × 700).

It will be seen by comparison with the previous figure that the Schmidt–Lanterman incisures were wider in the excised nerve than in the intact nerve. The incisures were originally seen in 1877 by Schmidt and Lanterman.

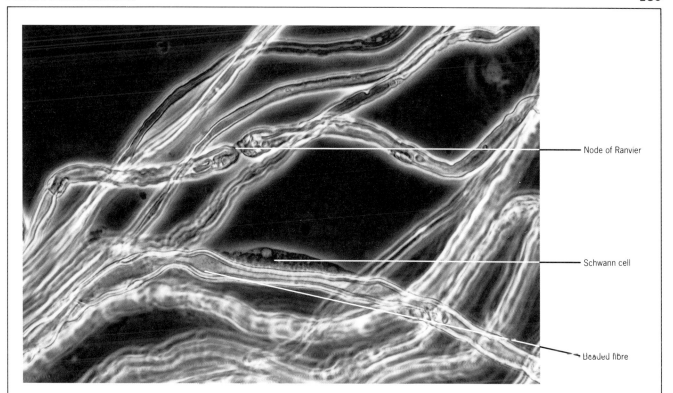

Figure 341 Teased 4-week-old rat sciatic nerve, to show myelinated nerve fibres and a Schwann cell (phase contrast, × 700).

Node of Ranvier

Schwann cell

Beaded fibre

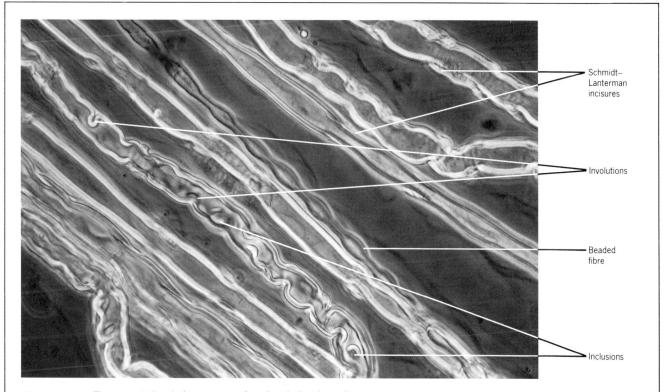

Schmidt–Lanterman incisures

Involutions

Beaded fibre

Inclusions

Figure 342 Teased rabbit sciatic nerve, to show beaded and myelinated nerve fibres and a Schwann cell (phase contrast, × 700).

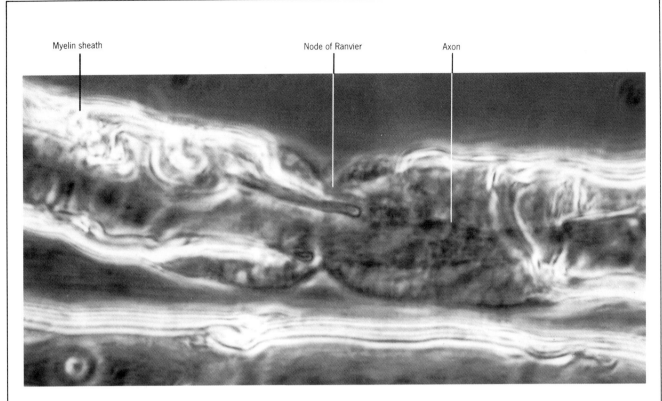

Figure 343   Isolated rabbit myelinated fibres from sciatic nerve, to show node of Ranvier (phase contrast, × 2000).

Note the central position of the axon.

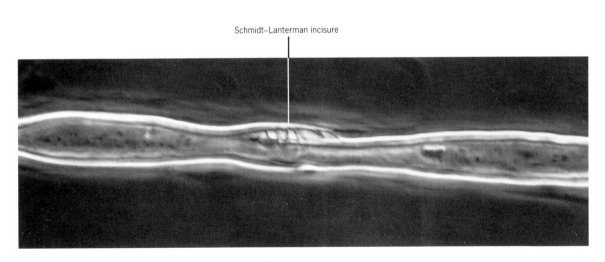

Figure 344   Isolated rat myelinated fibre from the sciatic nerve, to show Schmidt–Lanterman incisure on one side and intra-axonal particles (phase contrast, × 1300).

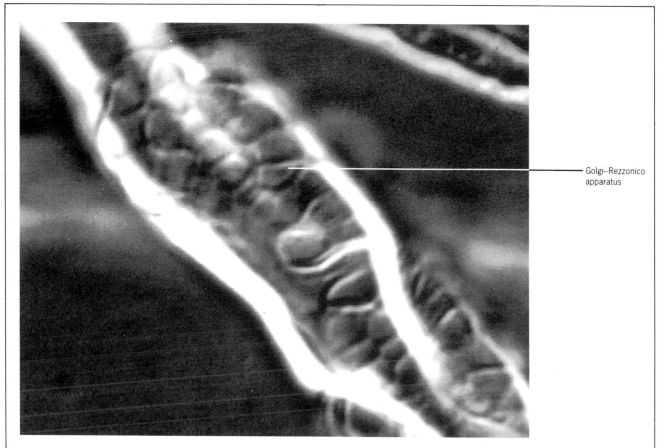

Golgi–Rezzonico apparatus

Figure 345 Isolated rabbit sciatic fibre, to show apparatus of Golgi–Rezzonico (Zeiss scanning differential interference contrast, × 4300). (By kind permission of Miss P. Gunter, of Zeiss Oberkochen.)

This was first reported in 1881 by Golgi.

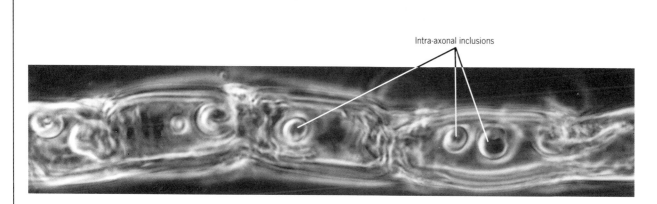

Intra-axonal inclusions

Figure 346 Isolated rabbit myelinated fibre from the sciatic nerve, to show intra-axonal inclusions (phase contrast, × 800).

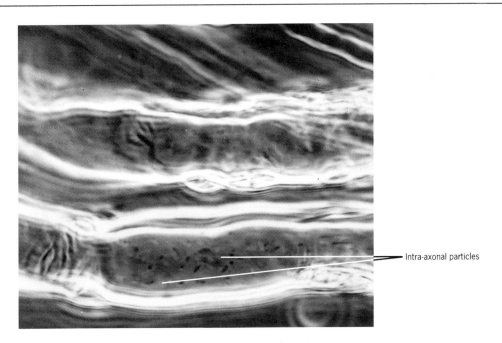

Figure 347   Isolated rabbit myelinated fibres from the sciatic nerve to show intra-axonal particles (phase contrast, × 1300). Particles can be seen moving in fresh axons.

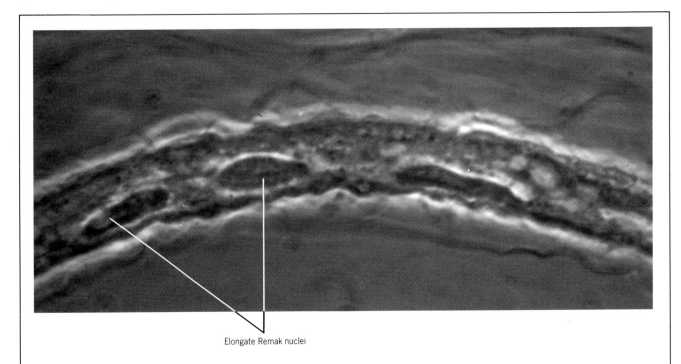

Figure 348   Isolated Remak fibre from rabbit sciatic nerve (phase contrast, × 2000).

Myelinated fibres

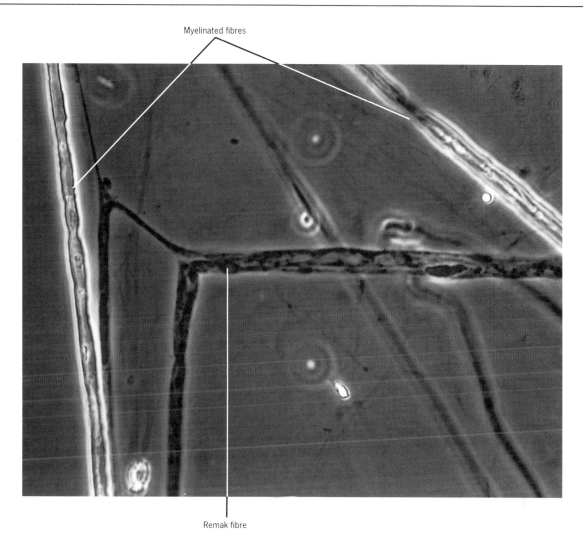

Remak fibre

Figure 349   Teased rabbit sural nerve to show myelinated and Remak fibres (phase contrast, × 800).

Note the branching of the Remak fibre.

SECTION

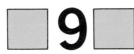

9

PITUITARY, PINEAL AND ADRENAL GLANDS

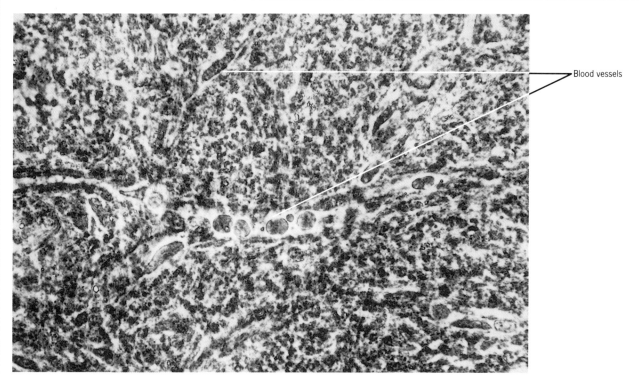

Figure 350   Unteased human posterior pituitary gland from a 73-year-old male, to show blood vessels *in situ* (phase contrast, × 700).

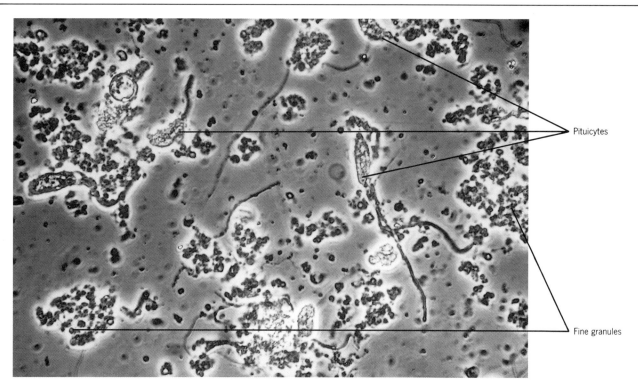

Figure 351   Isolated human pituicytes from the posterior lobe of a 73-year-old male; fine granules can also be seen (phase contrast, × 700).

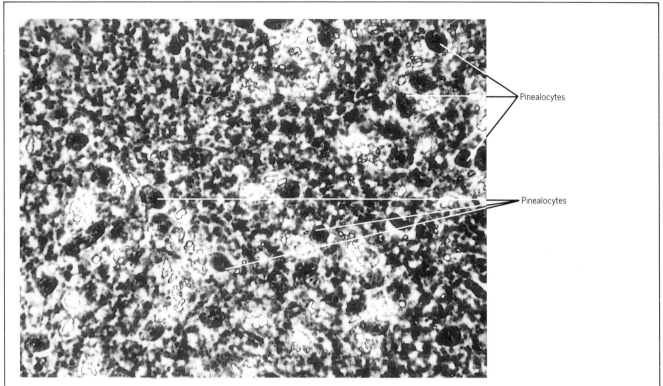

Figure 352 Thin slab of human pineal gland from a 66-year-old male, showing pinealocytes *in situ* (phase contrast, × 700).

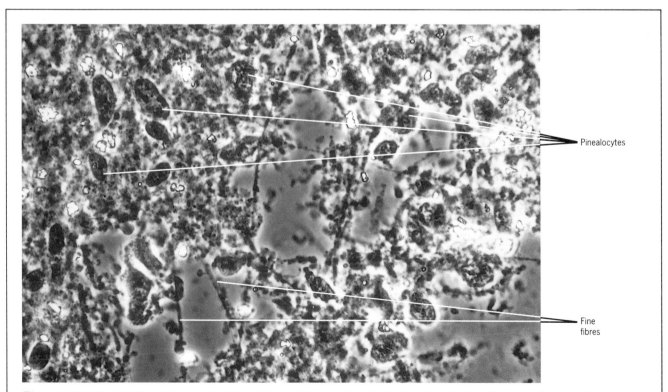

Figure 353 Partially teased human pineal gland from a 66-year-old male, to show pinealocytes, fine nerve fibres and fine granular material (phase contrast, × 700).

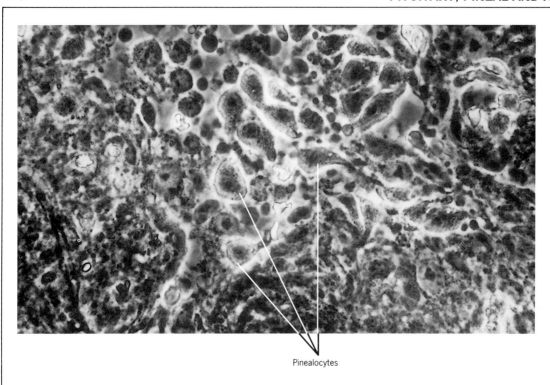

Pinealocytes

Figure 354   Partially teased guinea-pig pineal gland, to show pinealocytes (phase contrast, × 700).

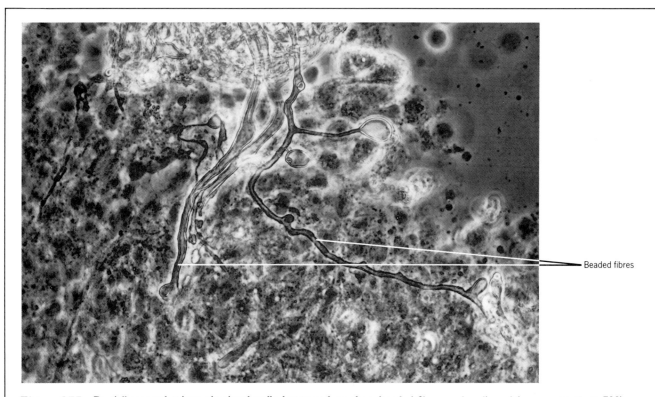

Beaded fibres

Figure 355   Partially teased guinea-pig pineal stalk, lower end, to show beaded fibres and endings (phase contrast, × 700).

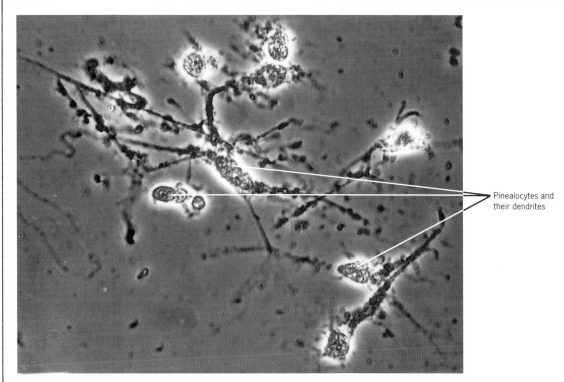

Pinealocytes and
their dendrites

Figure 356 Isolated human pinealocytes from a 66-year-old male (phase contrast, × 700).

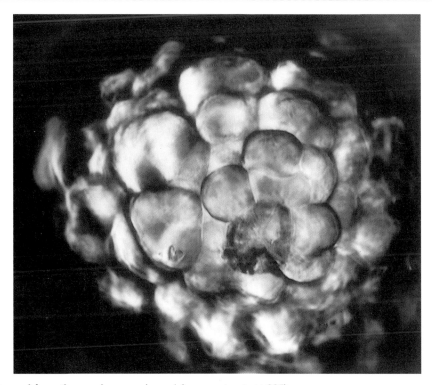

Figure 357 Brain sand from the previous specimen (phase contrast, × 335).

This is composed of the calcium salts, hydroxyapatite, laid down in lamellae. It provides a landmark for the position of the pineal gland in radiographs.

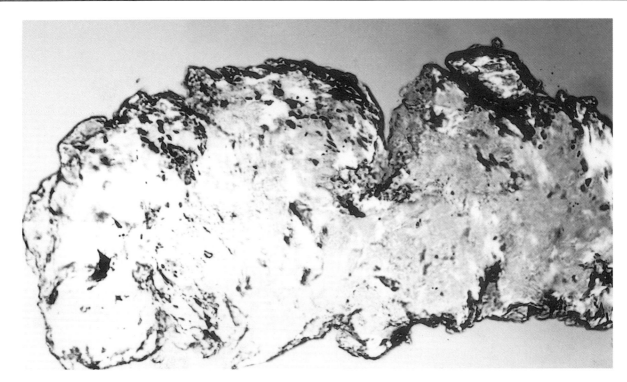

Figure 358   Another piece of human brain sand (bright field, × 800).

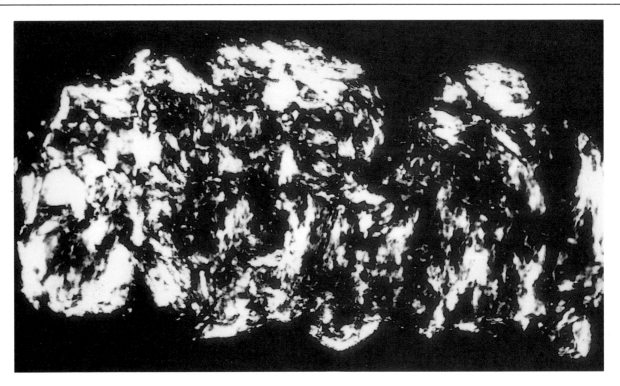

Figure 359   The same piece of brain sand as in the previous figure, but viewed through cross polars to show its birefringence (× 800).

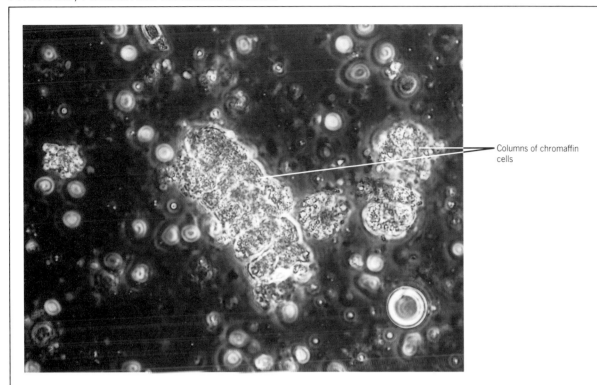

Figure 360   Partially teased rabbit adrenal medulla to show chromaffin cells in columns (phase contrast, × 700).

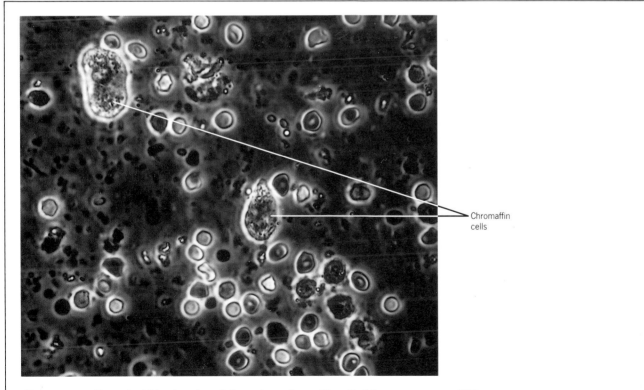

Figure 361   Teased rabbit adrenal medulla to show chromaffin cells (phase contrast, × 700).

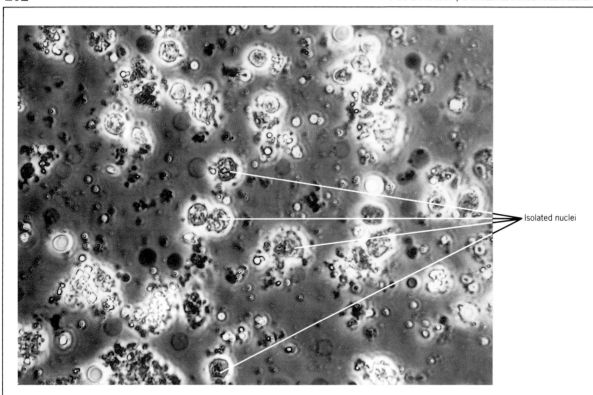

Isolated nuclei

Figure 362 Isolated nuclei and fine granular material from rabbit adrenal medulla (phase contrast, × 700).

SUMMARY OF THE STRUCTURE OF THE NERVOUS SYSTEM

The grey matter in fresh tissue appears brownish due to the presence of blood vessels, blood and neuron somas. Its main elements are neuron somas, dendrites, axons, neuroglial nuclei, beaded fibres, fine granular material and fine fibres. It also contains blood vessels of the different sizes, as do nearly all other tissues. A large proportion of the volume of grey matter is occupied by a fine granular material, which is frequently illustrated in this atlas. It may not have been seen before by light or electron microscopy, because it may have been washed out or extracted by the chemicals used in the staining and mounting procedures. The whole nervous system contains a network of fine dendrites or unmyelinated fibres, which are too thin and transparent to be seen, unless the surrounding tissue is stretched away from it.

The white matter consists of fibre tracts, large fibres, beaded fibres and droplets. The droplets and the beads in fibres vary in size and are translucent. They are found in freshly killed animal white matter, as well as in human post-mortem material, so that it is unlikely that they are fungi, bacteria, spores, or their products. Both the droplets and beads are shrunk or disappear as a consequence of staining and embedding procedures (Chughtai *et al.*, 1988). In life, they are obviously insoluble in the aqueous cellular fluids and tend to be spherical, so they may contain a high proportion of lipid.

The basal ganglia and the cranial nerve nuclei are intermediate between grey and white matter at the cellular level. They contain neuron somas, beaded fibres, fine fibres and fine granular material. Unidentified spherical cells with little cytoplasm and no dendrites can be seen occasionally.

The peripheral nervous system is dominated by myelinated nerve fibres with nodes of Ranvier. The Schmidt–Lanterman incisures are present in the living nerves, but are probably widened by manipulations of the tissue. Many axons are slightly invaginated and involutions can be seen within them. The peripheral nerves contain occasional Schwann cells with elongate nuclei on their periphery. Very fine fibres may be teased out, and it is impossible to know for certain whether they are nerve fibres or collagen fibres. Remak fibres appear black, and are very rare in cranial or peripheral nerves. No other unmyelinated fibres were seen.

APPENDIX

The effects of staining procedures on the appearances of rabbit medullary neuron somas. The micrographs **a**, **c** and **e** are of fresh neurons in normal saline. Micrographs **b**, **d** and **f** show the same neurons after staining with haematoxylin and eosin (**b**), Palmgren's procedure (**d**) and buffered osmic acid (**f**) (phase contrast, × 700). The bar is 50 μm. The shrinkages of the somas were to 22, 21 and 14 per cent, respectively, of the original areas (Chughtai *et al.*, 1987). (These photographs are reproduced by kind permission of the editor of *Microscopy* and the Quekett Microscopical Club.)

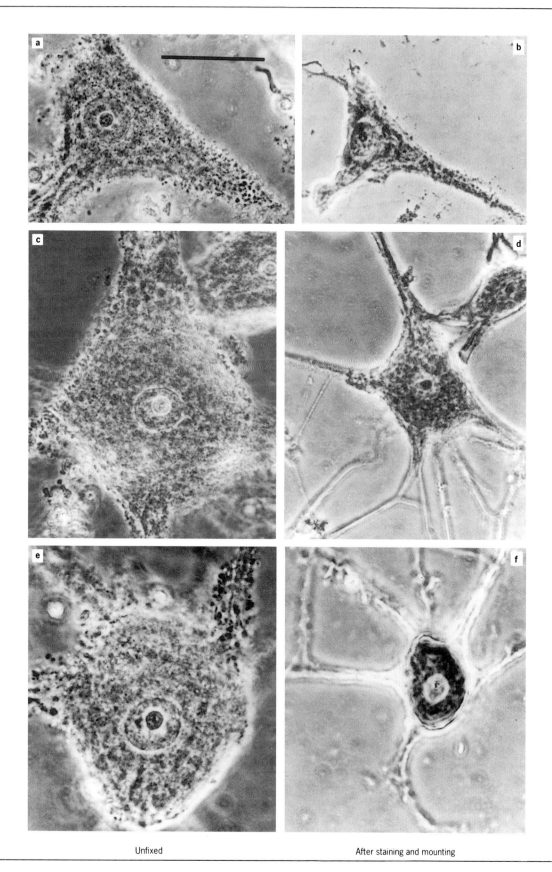

Unfixed

After staining and mounting

SELECTED REFERENCES

Baker, J. R. (1958). *The Principles of Biological Microtechnique*, p. 19. Methuen, London.

Betz, V. A. (1874). Anatomische Nachweis zwei Gehirncentra. *Zbl. med Wiss.* **12**, 578–580; 595–599.

Chambers, R. and Chambers, E. D. (1961). *Explorations into the Living Cell.* Commonwealth Fund, Harvard University Press, Cambridge, Massachusetts.

Chughtai, I., Hillman, H. and Jarman, D. (1987). The effect of haematoxylin and eosin, Palmgren's and osmic acid procedures on the dimensions and appearance of isolated rabbit medullary neurons. *Microscopy* **35**, 625–659.

Chughtai, I., Hillman, H. and Jarman, D. (1988). The effect of staining with haematoxylin and eosin, Golgi's stain and osmic acid on the appearance of single sciatic nerve and corpus callosal fibres of rat and guinea-pig. *Microscopy* **36**, 76–83.

Clarke, E. and O'Malley, C. D. (1968). *The Human Brain and Spinal Cord.* University of California, Berkeley.

Debus, E., Weber, K. and Osborn, M. (1983). Monoclonal antibodies specific for glial fibrillary acid (GFA) protein and for each of the neurofilament triplet polypeptides. *Differentiation* **25**, 193–203.

Dossel, W. E. (1966). Preparation of tungsten microneedles with a propane torch. *Stain Technol.* **41**, 61–63.

Ehrenberg, C. G. (1833). Nottwendigkeit einer feineren mechanischen Zerlegung des Gehirns und der Nerven vor der chemischen, dargestellt aus Beobachtungen von C. G. Ehrenberg. *Poggendorffs Ann. Phys.* **28**, 449–473.

Fernandez-Moran, H. (1952). The submicroscopic organization of vertebrate nerve fibres. *Exptl. Cell Res.* **3**, 283–359.

Golgi, C. (1881). Sulla struttura delle fibre nervosa midollate periferiche e centrali. *Arch. Scienze Med.* **4**, 221–245.

Gray, J. (1931). *A Textbook of Experimental Cytology.* Cambridge University Press, Cambridge.

Heilbrunn, L. V. (1956). *Dynamics of Living Protoplasm.* Academic Press, New York.

Hillman, H. (1986a). Hyden's technique of isolating mammalian cerebral neurons by hand dissection. *Microscopy* **35**, 382–389.

Hillman, H. (1986b). *The Cellular Structure of the Living Mammalian Nervous System.* MTP Press, Lancaster.

Hussain, T. S., Hillman, H. and Sartory, P. (1974). A nucleolar membrane in neurons. *Microscopy* **32**, 348–352.

Hyden, H. (1959). Quantitative assay of compounds in isolated fresh nerve cells and glial cells from control and stimulated animals. *Nature* **184**, 433–435.

Kuhne, W. (1862). *Uber die Peripherischen Endorgane der motorischen Nerven*, pp. 17–18. Englemann, Leipzig.

Lanterman, A. J. (1877). Uber den feineren Bau der markhltigen Nervenfasern *Arch. Mikroskop. Anul. Entwick. Mech.* **13**, 1–8.

Leeuwenhoek van, A. (1674). More observations from Mr. Leeuwenhoek. *Phil. Trans. Roy. Soc. B* **9**, 178–182.

Leeuwenhoek van, A. (1719). *Epistolae Physiologicae Super Compluribus Naturae Arcanis*, p. 312. Beman, Delft.

Meynert, T. (1872). The brain of mammals. In: (ed. Stricker, S., trans. Power, H.) *Manual of Human and Comparative Histology*, Vol. 2, p. 391. New Sydenham Society, London.

Obersteiner, H. (1903). Uber das hellgelbe Pigment in den Nervenzellen und das vorkommen weitere fettanlicher Korper im Centralnervensystem. *Arb. A. Neurol. Inst., Wein* **10**, 245–274.

Purkinje, J. E. (1838). Neueste Untersuchungen aus der Nerven und Hirn-Anatomie. *Bericht uber die Versammlung Deutscher Naturforscher und Arzte in Prag in September 1837,* pp. 177–180. Hasse, Prague.

Ramon y Cajal, S. (1892). Trans. Thorpe, S. A. and Glickstein, M. (1972). *The Structure of The Retina.* Charles Thomas, Springfield, Illinois.

Ranvier, L. A. (1871). Contributions à l'histologie et à la physiologie des nerfs peripheriques. *Compt. Hebd. Acad. Sci., Paris* **73**, 1168–1171.

Remak, R. (1836). Verlaufige Mitheilung mikroscopischer Beobachtungen uber den innern Bau der Cerebrospinalnerven und uber die Entwicklung ihrer Formelemente. *Arch. Anat. Physiol.* 145–161.

Remak, R. (1838). *Observationes Anatomicae et Microscopicae de Systematis Nervosi Structura* (thesis). Reimerionis, Berlin.

Sartory, P., Fasham, J. and Hillman, H. (1971). Microscopic observations of the nucleoli in unfixed rabbit Deiters' neurons. *Microsocopy* **32**, 93–100.

Schmidt, H. D. (1877). On the construction of the dark or

double bordered nerve fibres. *Month. Microsc. J.* **11**, 200–221.

Schwann, T. (1839). *Mikroscopisches Untersuchungen uber die Uebereinstimmung in der Struktur und dem Wachstum der Thiere und Pflanzen*, pp. 174–175. Reimer, Berlin.

Stilling, B. and Wallach, J. (1842). *Untersuchungen uber den Bau des Nervensystems*. Wigand, Leipzig.

Tellesniczky, K. (1898). Ueber die Fixierungs — (Haertung's) — Flussigkeiten. *Arch. Mikrosk. Anat.* **52**, 202–280.

De Vieussens, R. (1684). *Neuronographia Universalis*, pp. 55–56. Certe, Lyons.

Virchow, R. (1846). Uber das granulirte Ansehen der Wanderungen der Gehirnventrikel. *Allg. Z. Psychiat., Berlin* **3**, 242–250.

Virchow, R. (1856). *Gesammelte Abhandlungen Zur Wissenschaftlichen Medizin*, p. 890. Meidinger, Frankfurt.

Waldeyer-Hartz, H. W. G. (1891). Uber einige neuere Forschung im Gebiete der Anatomie des Centralnervensystems. *Deutsch. med Wschr.* **17**, 1213–1218.

Williams, P. L. and Hall, S. M. (1970). *In vivo* observations on mature, myelinated nerve fibres of the mouse. *J. Anat.* **107**, 31–38.

Zernike, F. (1934). Begungstheorie des Schneidenverfahrens und Seiner verbesserte Form der Phasenkontrastmethode. *Physica* **1**, 689–704.